YOGIC BLISS AND SEXUAL HEALING

AUTUMN NEEDLES

fanny*press*

Seattle, WA

Published by Fanny Press
PO Box 95462
Seattle, WA 98145

Cover design by Sabrina Sun

Contact: info@fannypress.com

ISBN: 978-60381-441-6 (Paper)

ISBN: 978-1-60381-442-3 (ePub)

Contents

Contents

Acknowledgments

I always wanted to write a book but I had no idea until I began how much work it was going to be. Thanks to all the people around me who tolerated my obsession while it was happening and had no doubt at all that I could finish what I started. A particular thanks to my partners just for being the wonderful people they are and supporting my work, but the biggest thanks has to go to my primary partner, Jamie, who had to live with me and put up with the fact that I did basically nothing during this time but sit in front of the computer in between running out to teach classes.

A special thanks to Russell Harmon for coming up with the term "cooperative pushing" and for allowing me to steal it from him. I expect I'll pay for it somehow.

And a thank you to all of my teachers along the way who influenced my thinking, in person or through their writing. I don't blame you for any mistakes I've made! Those are my own, and I take full credit for them.

Introduction

Stories

There are the stories we tell ourselves. There are the stories told about us. There are the stories told to us. When we meet, our stories meet as well, intertwining and mating, creating a whole new story. Which stories are true? I will try to tell the truth, but truly this is just another story.

When I was a little girl I was a voracious reader of fairy tales and Greek and Roman mythology. I loved being transported to other worlds through words and emerging at the end of the story wrung out and misty-eyed. I understood that the stories were make-believe, but I also wanted to find truth in them. I read anything I could find. At some point I realized many of the stories were told over and over again, but differently, running the gamut from sanitized happily-ever-after versions to older, crueler ones. I particularly remember when I first read *The Little Mermaid*, watching her journey onto land for the sake of love, giving up her beautiful voice and her family. She found her prince but received only pity and kindness from him, then watched in silence as he gave his love to a land-based girl. In her grief, she threw herself into the sea to drown, but was transformed into sea foam to ride the waves forever. How I cried! I was devastated to imagine that true love could be returned with pity, a life transformed and ended.

I was more devastated to compare the happy ending version of the story with the one I knew, and to realize that somewhere along the line the story itself had been transformed, sanitized into something easier and blander for the consumption of children. We children had been betrayed, I thought, but at least the betrayal was visible. Now that I knew, I could watch out for it.

My father introduced me to the Greek pantheon, reading me carefully chosen excerpts from the classic tales. I couldn't resist the stories, so I snuck back to the book and returned to the stories on my own, even though he forbade me to read them by myself. I soon found out why. These were not just the tales of love and valor I knew from his bedtime reading but also tales of rape and fear and murder, despair in the face of tragedy, betrayal of family and friends. Again, the truth beneath the offering was bigger and more complex than I had realized. For my protection, I had been given a lie. Or, at least, a partial truth. Children, I think, have a strongly developed sense of righteous indignation, without an understanding of how fragile they are, or that some truths need to be digested in smaller pieces. As a child all I saw was that I had been misled. Again.

In the fifth grade I sat in sex-ed, watching a movie about menstruation. The girls on the screen talked about how the bleeding only lasted a day or two, how sometimes there was discomfort, but never enough to disrupt their activities. How, despite the annoyance, it was a small price to pay to become a woman with the possibility of child-bearing in the future. I listened in outraged agony, arms clenched across my belly, pale and cramping and miserable, wondering if today would be a day when I overflowed and filled my chair with blood. What had I done to deserve this kind of protection from the truth? Was watching a friendly movie supposed to improve my experience, or was I being encouraged to toe the party line for the sake of the other girls?

One day after school, I remember my mother talking to me after I had been teased for something and was feeling sad and angry and hurt. She told me that sometimes it was better to look strong even when I felt weak, and that I should learn to control my reactions so no one would know how I really felt. She also suggested that it might be better for me to be more circumspect in what I told my friends, and that maybe some things were better left private. She wanted to protect me and give me tools to make my way in a sometimes difficult world. I appreciated her advice and followed it. It has served me well. Social ease makes life a lot more comfortable, and I got pretty good at it.

We all learn to do a certain amount of re-writing reality for the sake of ... something. Some of it is absolutely necessary. Think about how we learn things, layering information over time until we are able to think in more complex ways. For example, I think about learning about neurons, the cells of the brain and nervous system: In grade school it's enough to know that they act like little messengers, carrying around our thoughts and feelings. Later, we learn about the cells themselves, the parts that receive messages and the parts that send them on to the next cells. Much later, we learn about the specific chemistry and physics that make it possible for the membrane of the cell to transfer chemical and electrical information. It's not that we were lied to in grade school; we simply did not have the tools available to access and understand the whole picture.

Other kinds of re-writing can feel the same way, as though there are social tools we need in order to access particular personal information, but now we have other motives as well. We edit for the sake of ease, of clearing the way, of not making waves, of protecting people we care about, of protecting people we don't know, of fitting in with the crowd. I have participated in this type of re-writing my whole life, trying to protect myself, my family, my friends, the sensibilities of some faceless crowd. As a yogi (someone who studies and practices yoga), I try to follow the guidelines of the philosophy of yoga. One of those is satya, or truthfulness. However, I confess I have practiced evasion and misdirection when faced with simple questions in a public or work-related forum that required more

complicated answers than were expected or looked for.
People often use this type of evasion to connect in ways that
feel easy and familiar, to avoid hurting one another; there is
no scary ulterior motive. When someone at work asks me if I
am married or what my husband does for a living, they
certainly don't mean any harm, and, in fact, what they want
to do is connect with me. But when I know my answer isn't
the correct answer, I freeze. I know what people will be
comfortable hearing—what they want to hear—and it isn't
what I'm going to tell them. Then the truth feels awfully
slippery to me. I am caught between the desire for
connection and the desire for complete honesty. Frequently
we believe that the truth needs to be rearranged for some
greater good. We have a sense of what the truth is supposed
to be, and we try to rearrange ourselves around that. I know
I feel just a little twitchy, because I don't quite fit what ought
to be. I am afraid everyone else *does* fit, so we play a little
game of pretend.

I am pretty good at sliding under the radar and fitting in,
so my incentive to massage the truth in order to live
comfortably and easily is strong. This urge in myself to
magically transform my story is both frustrating and
fascinating, and I keep picking away at it like a scab that
hurts in a very interesting way yet requires healing. I am
drawn especially to an area of particular taboo—sex, how we
have it, how we want it, how it works and how it doesn't.
That's because I know that how I have sex, how I have
always *wanted* to have sex, does not fit the accepted mold.
But that just makes me curious—how many more of us are
there who don't fit the mold, but pass? Is there anyone really
in that mold at all?

We learn specific things about what we are supposed to
want and how we are supposed to communicate that want.
We are supposed to fall in love before we have sex, the
assumption being both that we will want to have sex before
we fall in love but will choose not to, and that when we fall in

10

love we will want to have sex with that person—and only that person—forever. Sex never needs to be defined because, in theory, we are all talking about the same thing when we speak of it. And we all want to do generally the same things when we have sex, right? We all want it to be special and meaningful, to take place with The One and to culminate in orgasm. We ought to have well-defined genders and desire the opposite gender from our own. If we are enlightened, we might understand that we could want someone of the same gender, but we are still supposed to do all of the other things the same way. We are supposed to communicate our desires romantically, but clearly. When we finally go to bed together, we are supposed to either just know what to do or communicate clearly and verbally what we really enjoy. We are not supposed to want sex before we reach a certain age. (Although it is understood that we are at the whim of our hormones, we are supposed to resist them!) We are supposed to communicate in a particular way, but we also learn a hidden language of sorts. If he does *this*, it means *that*. If she says *that*, it means *this*. There are books written about how to get a man, how to make a woman happy, how to keep a mate, how to spice things up ... but they never seem to involve much contemplation, either of our own reality or of the other person's. Societal values are assumed to equal the values of the individual, so we only get certain boxes to check off as options.

Climbing Out of the Box

I have a blog where I write about getting lost and finding my way, both literally and allegorically. I wrote in my blog one day about a time when I got together with two dear friends and celebrated Beltane, or May Day, with them. We were a little low energy (and it was raining), so we changed our original plans. Indoors instead of outdoors, short and sweet. Because we were all so low in energy we decided it would be a nice addition to give each other the May Day gift of sharing what we appreciate about each other. We are very different women who came together by chance, but over the years we have formed one of those bonds that you always hope will be a part of your life—a friendship where anything goes, where we can always speak the truth to one another. They each let me know that what they appreciate most about me is my direct communication, my willingness to be open about my life and my feelings (come what may), and that by so doing, I have let them in on a perspective they did not realize existed.

Years ago, when I attended my yoga teacher training, I heard the same thing from several of my fellow students there. One of the items I packed for my month at this training in Costa Rica was my vibrator. When my partner realized I was taking it along, she asked, "What will you say if they search your luggage and find it?" "I'll tell them I'm going to be away from home with no sex for a month! I've got to have something to entertain myself with." During the course of that month, sex was a big topic of conversation, probably because we were all away from home for a long time. I was very open about my own arrangements—that I had brought my vibrator and was unwilling to go without masturbating for a month, that I had more than one relationship, that pain and power were part of my sexual identity. Near the end of the month, one woman made a point of pulling me aside to tell me she was both surprised by and appreciative of my honesty, because it opened her mind to a different perspective.

I am humbled when I hear that, because I know that I still have so far to go in becoming completely open, completely honest. I look at all the places where I keep quiet, evade, go along to keep the peace, and I don't see enough honesty and forthrightness. On the other hand, I still struggle with how to go about doing all that in an ethical way. The kudos to me for what I have done so far just continue to remind me that I have so much further to go in becoming transparent. And this is the difficulty for me—how to become transparent and allow people to see me completely, while at the same time being respectful, doing no harm to others, and giving people space to draw away from what may frighten them. I want to live my life in the open, but I am also scared of what might happen if I am completely honest all the time. I don't always want to share everything with everyone all the time because I don't want to have to defend myself over and over again. It's easier sometimes to pretend to go along with everyone else. But then I have experiences like the ones described when I am completely honest, and I am pleasantly surprised by the response. Frequently I find that, while certainly not everyone is having my experience precisely, we are alike in the sense that we are all hiding something for some reason— from fear, from a desire to fit in, from duty, from a need to love and respect other beliefs and values around us. Do we really need to hide?

Two nights before that particular May Day celebration, my sweetie and I finally watched *Milk*, the movie about Harvey Milk, an openly gay politician who was murdered while in office. Honestly, I had avoided the movie a little because I knew how it ended and I did not want to mourn the loss again. But in watching it, I found myself looking back at my early days of coming out as a lesbian, and my discovery of my community, the history of those other gay men and lesbians who had become my people. My ancestors. I thought about the changes my partner and I have seen: twenty years ago we couldn't hold hands on the street without fear unless we were in the gay part of town. Now we do it almost without thought. And it is because of people like Milk who had the courage to allow themselves to be seen.

When you are gay or lesbian and begin to come out, you realize that the archetypal coming-out story is a myth in some ways, because it's always spoken of in the singular as though you do it once and you are done. The truth is you do it almost constantly, over and over again. After a while it gets exhausting, and you just want to go live your life and forget about it. Generally, we can all find a little corner to call our own and make our way in peace.

But I keep seeing little reminders all around me about why it is important to keep coming out. Our culture seems to have a strong desire to put everything and everyone into one big easily defined box. (Not to single out our culture; frankly, I think every culture does it. However, I only feel comfortable talking about the one I grew up in.) Once we have that box, there is a pervasive feeling that anyone who falls out of the box deserves whatever bad thing happens to them, and that it only happens to a few fringe people anyway, so why should we care? For the ones who know they don't live in the box, it can be terrifying and lonely. The funny thing is I think we all live outside the box and we just don't know it.

I honestly don't have a strong desire to share intimate details of my sex life with the world. I don't think it is anyone else's business what I do behind closed doors with other consenting adults, and I have a strong sense of privacy. I also think there is an appropriate time and place, both for being sexual and for talking about it. My desire for full disclosure does not mean talking about sex all day, every day, in every situation. That would be tedious and inappropriate. My life is bigger than what I choose to do in bed. But part of how I define myself as a human being, as a spiritual being, has a great deal to do with my sexuality. I don't want to erase that from my writing, or from my living, or from my teaching by presenting the sanitized Disney version of my life. Any child who has read *The Little Mermaid* and then watched the Disney version has the right to be furious over the betrayal of truth. Or if not to be furious, at least the right to see the difference and question it. We keep trying to force everything into the box, especially for kids, because we want them to believe that somehow all the confusions of youth smooth out and fall easily into line as we grow up, and everyone has a happy ending. Engaging with people who have checked a box in their minds when they meet me and try to relate to me from that perspective makes me squirm with discomfort. I am uncomfortable going along with them without speaking out, but I am also uncomfortable with making *them* uncomfortable by changing the terms of our social contract. I want an essay question, damn it, not a multiple choice question! I would like children (and adults who feel unhappy and trapped) to know that they don't necessarily need to check one of the pre-determined boxes, that they can choose something else. The only way I can see to do that is to live one of those choices openly.

We have so many methods in place to reinforce the box, to prop up the illusion of sameness. Every time I go to the doctor and check the box "single" under marital status, I erase myself a little. I am not single. It is a lie, but there is no place to state the truth about the web of relationships I live and love in on the form. I can explain and protest all I want, but that piece of paper remains implacable and unchanged, recording my life on paper as something it is not. Every time I allow assumptions to pass without comment, I help validate that box. I do it when I don't correct someone about the gender of my primary partner, or if I keep quiet and refuse to speak of the other partners in my life because it's just easier to talk about a spouse in the singular in everyone else's frame of reference. If I am honest about feeling prudish about bad language in songs piped over the overhead system at the gym, then someone may jump to the conclusion that I also share their other values. I am not telling the whole story. But who wants to live life always confronting or challenging everyone else, making them uncomfortable, when we really just want to get along, share space and engage?

Those experiences make me even more aware of the accomplishments of the people who came before me. My family strongly emphasizes family ties and family history, and my mother has often exhorted me to remember and honor them in making my life choices. I don't think she realizes that I tend to think less about my blood relations who made my physical existence possible than about the historical people I discovered along the way—those who lived their lives with so much honesty and visibility that I was able to find them and follow their teachings. Somehow they managed to check off the "none of the above" box to show me and others a way out of the narrow options we've been given ... to let us know that we can live and breathe outside the box and still be happy.

Back to that blog. I began writing it because I had noticed that my truly abysmal sense of direction had allowed me to have several interesting and educational experiences, which came about through getting lost fairly spectacularly over and over again. I recognized I had a tendency to wander about aimlessly and get lost metaphorically in life as well. So I thought it might be wise to examine that quality and make peace with it, learn where it had something of value to offer. Because my yoga practice is a lens through which I view my experience, I often look to yogic principles to make sense of things. When I first began writing this as a post to my blog, I thought it was connected to the yogic principle of satya, truthfulness. After watching the movie *Milk*, I returned to my writing with the feeling that I was actually writing about ishvara pranidhana, surrender to the Lord. The Lord in yoga is understood as a pure divine awareness, as Stephen Cope puts it in *The Wisdom of Yoga* "...the Witness behind the Witness." Cope understands the concept of the Lord as being almost a gravitational force that draws us in. In yoga we work to align ourselves with it, the idea being that we can't resist gravity anyway, so if we can be aware of it and align with it, we can let go of resistance.

16

I think initially it can be confusing, all this talk of resistance and surrender in connection with real life. Because am I not being resistant by being so stubborn and contrary about forcing the truth of my life in sight of others? And can't I surrender by just being quiet and going along with the status quo? Here is the problem with that: it is not the Box we need to surrender to, but the Lord. The Box is something that is constantly created and shored up by fearful people—myself included. Its purpose is to control, understand and quantify something too big to control, understand and quantify. People like Harvey Milk understood that we need to surrender to the truth of our own lives, to live them out in the open and transparently, understanding and accepting that there will be consequences we can't control, but that we must surrender to that larger force. We can become the ancestors, showing a way out of despair for those who can't find the right box to check, until finally we all understand that there is no box.

Me and My Body

When I was little, I loved to dance. And I loved to read. That was all I really wanted to do—dance and read. I've already talked about reading, about that sense of losing myself in other worlds. Dancing felt like something very precious and fragile—journeying in my body to a place out of time where I could be free. I was shy about it and unwilling to commit my love for it into the open air where anyone could see. I was afraid it would be taken from me or that I wouldn't be good enough, not worthy of its gift. Sometimes I would sit on the edge of my bed and just breathe, feeling the delicate wings of joy quivering within me. I was scared to move lest I startle it away, but I needed to release it somehow. It was too large for me to just hold inside. Only dancing could set it free to fly with me. I was afraid, though, that if people saw my joy, they would kill or imprison it, make fun of it, something. I wasn't sure, but I knew it would be taken from me.

At the same time, I already had a sense that there might be other activities I could do with my body that might let my joy out to play with me. I was not sure of all that was available to me with this body, but I was beginning to get a few ideas. I had a huge family of stuffed animals, seven of whom shared my bed every night. One in particular, Panda (who was, of course, a panda bear), was my special favorite, although I tried not to let the others know. I had already begun exploring my private parts with my fingers, tracing the folds, noticing how differently each piece responded to touch. Because I did read a lot, I knew a little bit about orgasms. A very little bit. I had tried to get information as best I could from the dictionary, but the dictionary defines things in circular ways. In order to know what one word means, you need to know what all the other words mean that define it. So my grasp was still vague.

One morning I woke up with Panda between my legs. I began to rub against his fur. It felt good. A kind of pressure was building, as though things were getting a little too large inside. I didn't know exactly what an orgasm was but I wanted to feel one. I was also scared of it. The feelings that arose when I rubbed against Panda felt so large as to be overwhelming. I couldn't really even define them as pleasure because they were too big for that word. It would have been like saying I liked to dance. I didn't like dancing; I *had* to dance, I was made to dance, the dance needed me to live it. It wasn't a question, it was an emphatic declarative. This other was no question, either, but I did know enough to recognize a dividing line when I saw one. On this side was me, a girl child; on the other ... well, I wasn't sure, but I knew it was a whole different reality over there.

Over the years I continued my sexual relationship with my body. (Yes, my first orgasm was with Panda, thanks for asking.) Panda was my first, but my curiosity extended out to, well, pretty much everything. I wanted to make everything sexual, or maybe it was more that everything *felt* sexual. Everything became a tool to explore my sexuality. I masturbated with Barbie and found that, while her foot provided an interesting protrusion to rub on my clit, her hair was an exciting texture to feel brushing my labia. I noticed how nice the little feet of flies felt on my arm, so I tried to coax them to land and walk on my sex. I loved the way my body felt and I was curious about everything to do with it. I even tried looking at my various fluids under a microscope to see what was there.

I also hated certain things about my body and tried to change them. As I hit puberty, I often felt betrayed by my body, like it had become a whole different creature—unfamiliar and inimical to me. I divided it into parts, choosing the parts I liked (my legs, for example! I would put on pantyhose and pose to admire them) and the parts I didn't (my sloping shoulders, getting too much attention from grown-ups determined to make me stand up straight). I would study my face endlessly in the mirror, covering half at a time to make myself into two completely different people based on the asymmetry of my features. Then I would resent putting my glasses on over the results. As I grew up, I did what we all do to some degree—separated myself from my body as a whole, developing certain beliefs about the landscape of my physicality, while absorbing the rights and wrongs of my family and the culture around me as to what was appropriate to do with my body.

I knew what I wanted to do with it. I wanted to have sex. And I wanted to dance. I wanted to do both with abandon, without fear. I couldn't quite figure out how to do that, so I allowed my fear to have the deciding vote for a long time. Fear of being hurt, physically or emotionally. Fear of what people might think. Fear of what my mother would think. Fear of leaving the path of an ordinary life.

* * *

I was at a restaurant the other night, seated next to a family with a little girl who was about four years old. Frankly, she drove me crazy, wiggling all over and around her chair. I don't think she was still for a single moment. But because she captured my attention—mostly because I was scared she'd knock over our water glasses—I was really watching her carefully. I realized that she inhabited her body so cleanly, filling herself up to all her edges; there wasn't a piece of her that seemed disconnected. She was lacking awareness, which is, I think, what we gain as we grow older, but she had that animal sense of herself. I couldn't help but think about what will happen to her as she grows up, what may be happening to her already, skewing her perspective of her own landscape, creating layers of thought and ideas and experience around her natural physicality, taking her farther and farther out of touch with that naïve body intelligence she was born with. The forces that come to bear on the sense we have of ourselves can be blatant or subtle. I don't think we can point to just one that ultimately creates our belief around the body. So, I look at this little girl and I don't know. When she looks at the world around her, what does she see reflected back? What does she learn from billboards and magazines, from the pretty pictures since she can't read yet? What is she learning from her parents, either what they explicitly tell her or what she reads from their responses and behaviors? What is she learning from her own experiences with her body, in private or with others? Then there are the parts we don't like to talk about. Is there someone close to her, taking advantage of her innocence and changing her world forever? I'm calling her a girl because a girl is what I see, but does she feel easy in that gender, or is she already wondering how things went wrong? Such a small body to withstand such forces, as we all must do, as we all have done.

And sex! Don't get me started on all the beliefs we pile on sex! (Whoops! Too late ...) Sex is dirty and wrong. Sex should only be done with someone you love and who loves you. Sex is for making babies. Sex is a beautiful natural thing. Sex is a male penis in a female vagina. Sex is scary. Sex is private. Sex is naughty. Sex is painful. Sex shouldn't hurt. We learn that sex should never be talked about openly, and yet many social situations involve a lot of heavy sexual innuendo that we are supposed to be able to navigate. And because sex is a physical activity relating to the body and specifically to the unmentionable parts of the body, we are supposed to keep it private. At the same time, we are supposed to be able to switch that off and become uninhibited in discussing every detail with our lovers and our doctors. Something about this doesn't add up for me.

Somehow other elements come in to pollute our experience so we become alienated from ourselves, setting up layers of rules and protections and beliefs around our bodies. We are supposed to renounce the body or beat it into shape. It is shameful and dirty. It produces waste we're embarrassed by and changes shape over time in ways we can't always control. We are supposed to hide it. We are also supposed to love it and give it pleasure and not be ashamed of it. So which is it? Do we talk about it or don't we? What are we supposed to do with this walking, talking creation?

I don't have answers to all of those questions. In fact, what I mostly have are questions of my own. I am not interested in talking about the right or wrong of how we are socialized and what we learn from it. I'm not really even interested in how we ought to be doing it, because I don't have confidence that my own answer would fit everyone's needs. Even in my own head, I go around and around in circles trying to figure out what would be ideal. I am more interested in peeling off the layers, and—once we develop that self-awareness—looking more closely at ourselves. For me personally that observation involves using the principles of yoga as my lens. As an adult I look back and see my body as the home I was born into and understood intuitively to a large degree. Whatever I didn't understand became my playground to explore and get to know. I believe that my body was designed as a conduit for joy, for play—child play that expanded into adult play. "Play" meaning a special time apart from the other realities of life. A time for imagination, for exploring emotional range, for expanding ability, for a connection with the world around me, including, or maybe *especially* including, other people. A time to learn to communicate—to ask and to receive, creating a safe space to step into the unknown with another. I believe that making use of the body in this way is the right thing to do.

What's It All About, Anyway?

So now you're wondering, what on earth kind of book is this, anyway? So far, she's dithered on about yoga and masturbating and bodies and getting lost—where is she going with this? You have to remember my lousy sense of direction—I even have to find my way into my own book. There is no clear path laid out before me; getting lost and finding the way back are part of the journey. Finding and recognizing truth, communicating it to ourselves and others, knowing when to explore it and expose it and when to protect it or leave it: I can't see a simple way to get there.

Partly this is me thinking out loud, speaking my own truth in my own stories, in the hope that others out there will either see themselves and feel seen and witnessed by a stranger or feel that they have permission to speak the truth in turn. My writing is, in some way, the full disclosure I wish I could make in every social situation. My guess is that, while my socially challenging and taboo parts are different in some ways from yours or hers or his, we all have them. And we all hide them. I hope that this book is helpful to people trying to find their own way through the layers around them, creating their own personal map to truth. It is easy to look around and feel lonely because it looks like everyone except you is living in a very particular way, walking that clearly marked path, and that you have to keep your secret because you won't be accepted otherwise. Each secret is a little different, but I don't believe we are really all that different at heart. We are all learning to be in the world the best way we can.

Because this book is me speaking from my experience, it is skewed to my interests. I work with my body and I play with my body. My work involves helping people find physical health and learning to use their bodies better. My play involves things like dancing and taking walks, but it also to a large degree involves sex and sexuality. Body image, body health, and physical intimacy with others are all areas where I see strong assumptions and beliefs as well as strong taboos, so those are the topics most interesting to me personally. I see so much discomfort around those areas that those are the areas I am most drawn to discuss. Discomfort and taboos perk up my ears and send me sniffing around. Bodies and sex are exciting and interesting to me. I want everyone to be happy and healthy in their bodies and their sexuality.

What This Book is Not

This is not a how-to book about sex or yoga. I'm not going to talk about sex tips to spice up your relationship, or how to tie each other up, or safety concerns about sexually-transmitted disease, or yoga poses that promote better sex. There are many resources available on all of those topics.

This is not erotica or pornography. While I write about some of my experiences in very explicit language, I am not writing with the intention to titillate. If my writing is used in that way, it's fine with me. Whether my book ends up on the nightstand in a stack of mysteries and biographies or tucked under the bed with the pages falling easily open to some well-loved story is all the same to me. My main purpose is to write truth. It's just that sometimes truth is sexy.

This is not my autobiography or memoir. I am much more interested in a dialogue than a monologue. My hope is that some of my thoughts and experiences can illuminate a path for others. I know that I have been deeply and profoundly changed and helped by reading what others have written, if for nothing else than a little shift in perspective. If I can create a tiny bit of that for other people, I will be satisfied.

This is not a book about relationships, alternative or otherwise. I am polyamorous and kinky and queer, so that is my frame of reference, but the book is not about that or about navigating those realms. If you have questions about those areas specifically, I have included a resource list in the back, with books that have been helpful to me.

Why Yoga?

I mentioned that dance is my joy, but dance doesn't come with a spiritual philosophy attached to it. Yoga, on the other hand, does. Lots of people think of yoga as a physical exercise. That is one aspect of it. It is also a philosophy, a spiritual tradition, a way of approaching life. In this book, that is the aspect I will be using and discussing to some extent. Yoga has been particularly helpful in integrating all the different parts of myself, including my sexuality. If you want the physical poses, this is the wrong place to find them. If you want a detailed rundown of the philosophical aspects of yoga, this is also the wrong place to find that. Here, I use yogic philosophy as a context or a viewing lens. I will talk about some aspects of yoga explicitly, but often I will just use them as a tool to talk about other things. I hope it makes you hungry to find out more. Maybe I'll see you in class some day. When I use a term from yoga, I will define it in the text.

I have structured the book around a particular concept in yoga concerning the layers, or sheaths, of the self. The book has five parts, corresponding with the layers of the self we talk about in yoga: the physical body, energy, thought and emotion, the witness, and bliss. The layers of the book, just like the layers of the self, are not easily teased apart. There is overlap and echoing among the different pieces. What I hope is that some part of that will speak to you, either to validate your own experience and embolden you to live from the truth in your heart, or to give you food for thought, a window into a different way of being, or permission to be true to your desire.

What About the Sex?

There is some of that in the book, and what there is, is explicit. I use my own experience for illustration throughout. I draw from my life because my ideas are drawn from my own experiences. All of us need to take ideas and test-drive them with our own experiences to see how valid or useful those ideas are. While I could take 100 interviews and boil them all down to something statistically significant, the truth is, you would still need to make the final determination of validity for yourself. While there may be people in my life who recognize themselves here, I have changed or left out names and some details in the stories. I can't make the choice for anyone else whether to stay anonymous or not.

Because I am using my own sexuality and sexual experiences as the examples in this book, the perspective is also from my end of the sexual arena. I have identified for most of my life as either bisexual or lesbian or queer, and my relationship structure was monogamous for thirteen years. Then I became polyamorous, which means I have multiple people in my life whom I love and with whom I have sex. I am kinky, which means that some of the sex I talk about falls outside what many people think of as sex. My intention is not to exclude other experiences or to invalidate them. These are just my experiences, and they are the only things I can speak of with any authority. I don't think anyone "ought to" live my life; I think everyone "ought to" live whatever life is right for that individual. I also don't think there is anything bad or shameful or wrong about my way.

I occasionally use some terms regarding sex and sexuality that are not in common use, so I will define them here. BDSM is short for several couplets: bondage and discipline, dominance and submission, and sadism and masochism. BDSM is a type of activity, sexual or not, covering a lot of territory and involving some sort of pain or power or a lot of rope. Within the BDSM community, we talk about our activities as "play." Generally, there is a Top, who functions like the lead in dance, calling the shots, as well as a Bottom, who functions more like the follow in dance, receiving the sensation and responding to it. A Scene is a planned sexual or BDSM encounter that is negotiated in advance. Polyamory means what it sounds like—having multiple loves. When I talk about my partners, I am talking about the people I love and with whom I share my life in some way.

My stories are intended as illustrations, but I hope they are also hot and fun sometimes, or silly and thought-provoking at others, or uncomfortable, or familiar. Whatever they are to you, I hope you allow yourself to use them at least to practice being a witness. Because they are my stories, you will be a witness to my experiences rather than your own, but I hope you accept them as an invitation to spend some time with whatever emotions or thoughts or responses you have. Take the time to sit with whatever they bring up and don't be shy; feel free to use them as you choose. Sometimes it's easiest to practice being a witness to a stranger's experience. I'm not in the room with you as you read, to judge you for what you feel. Sometimes even as I write I can feel an urge to pull away from what I'm writing, to pretty it up, or change it in some way. It scares me to make myself vulnerable and exposed, not just to you, but to myself. It is not always easy to look myself in the face and say, "I know you." But this is what we practice—sitting with truth.

I am interested in how we touch one another, whether through our words and actions, or literally, physically. I think there is a way to tap into the body's own intelligence, and then teach it to work smarter, to use its body sense. If we can learn to do that, maybe we can also learn to be more observant when we say things like, "I need" or "I want." I want to talk about sex and sexuality, how they happen, what we think about them, what we do with them. Talking about sex means talking about connecting with other people and how that happens—whether we're having sex with them or just trying to connect in an honest way. We don't live in a bubble. The more we can figure out ourselves and each other, creating space for the truth of who we are, the better off we'll be.

Context

"Open your mouth ... wider ... just as wide as you can get it. Stick your tongue out." I'm panting, hungry, looking up at him, his face partly covered by the camera he's holding. I sneak a glance at his cock as he pulls it out of his fatigues, over the top of his underwear, and shudder away again. I haven't had an actual male penis in my mouth for twenty years. Later, watching the film, I laugh at myself going cross-eyed as I peek up at it. Now my mouth is open and I can't see his cock anymore; it's too close to me. Then I feel it, silky and warm on my tongue, the head is past my teeth and I have his cock in my dry mouth. "I'm going to make you gag ... more."

Roll the tape back. "Suck my big fat cock. Oh yeah." Really, it's my big fat cock, purchased at Babeland, the black version of Adam #3, strapped onto her hips, but that's a technicality. I'm wearing the lipstick that dries solid so it won't wipe off—my cocksucker lipstick, I joke—so she can enjoy watching my red lips wrapped around her cock while I struggle to take it deeper. My fist is deep in her cunt.

And back again. I have never sucked a strap-on silicone cock before. At first the idea seemed strange, alien even— what's the point of sucking something that can't feel?—but my curiosity has grown. And now I'm eyeing her cock over the spanking bench and right at this moment it's the tastiest thing I've ever seen. I want it in my mouth so badly. I'm crawling over the bench to get to it and she teases me. "Is this what you want?" She grabs my hair and pulls me forward.

Again, further back. I'm in the basement with my boyfriend. He is lying on the couch, one arm thrown over his face, one hand on the back of my head. I feel bold. I've pulled his cock out of his jeans and am learning its shape with my tongue. This is the first time I have been brave enough to take the initiative and try something I have been dreaming of. We hear footsteps on the stairs and he scrambles to sit up while I drape myself over his lap as casually as I can to greet his father who has come down to chat with us.

And once more. "No, Sam, no! No please. No." "Just suck my dick and I'll take you home. C'mon. No big deal." I don't know what else to say. The only word I have is no, and it's not working. I am sixteen years old and so is he, I think, or maybe seventeen. He is a friend, and I don't understand how we've ended up here, parked in an unfamiliar field, after he offered me a ride home. I keep trying to superimpose that word "friend" on what is happening here, aware that my very lack of awareness of my surroundings has put me in danger, and still trusting to his friendship to get me eventually back home. I have his cock in my mouth and it's completely unreal. I keep hearing, "Sweet sixteen and never been kissed," over and over and over in my head. It's somewhat true. The only kisses I've had so far were snuck back when I was twelve years old—awkward, inappropriate things. And now I have a boy's penis in my mouth when all I want is for him to let me go home. I think I've jumped a few bases. While I am struggling to just get through this so I can go home, I am also very aware that this is my first blowjob. It feels like it's written in capitals across my brain with a self-important space between each word. My Very First Blowjob. This is the beginning of all of those first times in sex. New parents have their baby books: Baby's first shoes, first solid food, first steps, first words. I will never make a scrapbook of it, but I recognize a new entry in my own book of firsts: My First Blowjob. It's not at all how I would have wanted it, but it's the first time, so even as I am rising out of my body to escape it, at the same time I want to be good at it. This is what girlfriends are gauged by, if my reading of porn and the questionnaires in women's magazines is at all accurate. And is he actually going to come in my mouth? I've heard about the big "spit or swallow" debate, and I'm not sure what to do when it happens. I am trying to get away from it, block it out, stop it. And I am trying to remember every piece of it. It's not supposed to be this way. But this is the way it is.

So is this really the first thing I want you to know about me? The story of my life through the blowjobs I've given? All that high-minded philosophy about truth-telling and surrender to the Lord has brought us to this? It's a little crass, isn't it? This book is not the story of my life, through blowjobs or otherwise. But it is a book about being honest about sex, and I suppose it is appropriate that it begins with me being honest about my sex.

In a way, though, this is exactly the right way to begin, because it encapsulates all of the ideas I want to talk about. I want to talk about how sex really happens, about how we define it and about how it defines us. How when we talk about desire, we are also talking about fear and the unknown, the separation between fantasy and reality. We are talking about context. We are talking about what happens to our bodies and about how our energy flows. We are talking about boundaries, holding them solid, respecting them, having them destroyed or damaged, pushing up against them purposefully. We are talking about inspiration, creativity. Consent, or the lack of it. Taboo. We are also talking about communication, since sex is a kind of conversation. We are talking about limitations of time and space, getting exactly what we want or being frustrated by never getting what we want. We are talking about bodies in all of their raunchy uncomfortable glory—how we feel about them and what we do with them together. And we are talking about change over time.

Should I be trying to use better, nicer language in my descriptions? But no. If I'm going to sit down and talk about sex, I might as well talk about my real experiences in language that is comfortable for me. Not about what I learned in sex-ed. Or about what I learned as a child from friends and family or from the culture around me, my peers—what I am supposed to do and what is allowed. Or maybe I want to talk about all of that, too. Maybe there's no way around it. I want to sit with the idea of sex long enough to peel off those layers of belief and expectation, because they are part of my experience, too. Peel them off and see what's underneath. Who am I really and what do I want? I want to feel safe enough to look at what is desired, at what I desire, so that I (we) can be informed by it, guided by it, without being blindly compelled by it. I want to find the space between "I want/I have to/I'm supposed to" and action. Sit with it a little bit and get familiar with the difference between "want" and "should."

My lack of a sense of direction has made me extra sensitive to other aspects of my landscape, both internal and external. Because I don't have an innate sense of direction, I have to examine and question everything in order to find my way. Maps are imbued with a mystical quality for me. They are my sacred objects and I need them to be accurate. I trust them to guide me. They help me feel safe in an uncertain world. On the other hand, when I find out a map is inaccurate, I feel lost and betrayed. When you think about it, a map is a kind of story we tell ourselves about the land around us. Different types of maps tell different stories, and the accuracy of the map depends on the ability and the integrity of the mapmaker. In some ways, I think about my body and my sexuality this way—as territory to be mapped. I want to do it carefully and accurately so that I can be safe as I find my way.

In yoga we talk about the layers, or sheaths, of ourselves. The first layer is the physical body, the second is the energy body, and the third is our thinking/feeling body. We can imagine a child being born, the physicality of being propelled out into the world and being forced to draw that first breath of air, to bring in energy from the outside with no intermediary for the very first time. As the child grows, thoughts and feelings come over time, first just as themselves, then the words to match the thoughts and feelings and talk about them. Our goal in yoga is to link all of these sheaths together, to let them work as a unit to reduce the chatter among the different parts that are each trying to go their own way. Having unified them into a whole, we can begin to recognize a fourth layer, the inner witness. The witness is that untouchable part—whole and perfect and watching every experience from a safe place. Once the witness is accessible we have the opportunity to experience the fifth layer, which is bliss. The fifth layer is always a part of us, but we are usually unaware of it until our witness awakens to recognize that we live in the possibility of never-ending perfect joy—independent of our mood, our thoughts, our physical health, what everyone else is doing, or our status. Bliss is already a part of the landscape.

In the first layer, we look at the body and its geography. Let's do a little digging, down through the layers of history and connection to find the different voices of the body and the different ways we relate to it. The earthiness of the body leads me to think about safety and security, a solid foundation and strong connection with the earth. When I think about my own first experiences with mapping my sexuality, safety and security are not concepts that feel natural. Instead, what I can see is the beginning of taboo, marking off territory that is off limits and scary, not allowed, becoming more fascinating over time. I can see in my own history the beginnings of my eroticizing want/don't want, this push/pull between something that feels wrong or bad but that is also exciting in some way. The fear of being found out. And maybe recognizing what belongs to me, what I can define as mine to protect my health and safety. Once we define boundaries, put stakes in the ground to say, this right here is safe and known and that out there is scary and unknown (but also inviting), we can start to explore. Isn't that how so many fairy tales play out, by having someone venture outside the known and get into trouble? Sex wouldn't be as fun if we took all the adventure out of it. Frequently, though, an unsafe culture of sex exists around us. We need to make or find a safe space for ourselves to explore exactly those things that frighten us or that we are uncertain about. We can then be explorers of the unknown. We can begin by looking at what we think we know about our bodies and how we think about them, then maybe peel that away and question the validity of our knowledge by paying attention to what is really there. At the root of things, we are beginning already to develop a witness consciousness, observing ourselves with benevolent curiosity so that we can begin to create that sense of care for ourselves.

Once we begin to examine the actual territory of ourselves, we can start drawing new lines, creating an accurate map. The act of observing ourselves creates energy that we can learn how to use. We figure out our priorities, directing our energy in particular directions and closing it off in others, or feeling our energy drawn in certain ways. When we begin to draw a map, we want to share it, overlap it with someone else's and exclaim over the places we've each been—the places we may want to discover together. We feel desire for the other. We can begin to define what we want and what we don't want, so that we are pulled toward certain things and away from others. Yoga is often about balancing two opposite forces to create an even flow. One balance is the one between effort and surrender. We have to learn how to direct our desire and let go of it at the same time while holding solidly at the center. We awaken to an understanding of our own power. In order to be powerful, do we need to try to overwhelm someone else or can we learn to allow their personal power as well? How do we grow our hearts, our courage in order to actually step out and engage with the world sexually? Who are all these others out there and how do we play well together?

We are already starting to think about everything, to feel an emotional connection to certain people or certain activities. Our energy spills out into thoughts and feelings, and we're into the third layer. Maybe with the body we were looking at the geology of ourselves. Now we can be archaeologists, examining the layers of education we've received from our peers, our religion, our family, and our schools. When we see those new exciting places open on the horizon, we need ways to communicate them. We need to

find a voice for this body of ours, to communicate where our
energy is flowing, what we think and feel. How do we
communicate with others about sex? We have all kinds of
ways of talking with one another. What are our fantasies
and, when we begin to share them with others, how do we do
that ethically and in good faith? We can begin to examine
our thoughts and feelings about sex more carefully through
our fantasies and our actual experiences. We may find that
we edit reality for ourselves without even knowing it,
working our way around areas of taboo or blind spots in our
vision, or we may find ourselves stuck in patterned
responses. As we connect with others, we look for a way to
do that respectfully, bringing them into our circle of
observation. At the same time they become a witness for us,
helping us see ourselves through different eyes. We begin to
define things more clearly. We learn to make space for what
we think and feel without fighting what is hurtful or feels
bad, without following blindly where our thoughts lead us.
We learn to play with what we have available to us.

Having placed our will in a particular direction, can we
surrender into whatever comes, knowing that we live with
limitation? What is the purpose of what we choose to do?
Are we being effective in doing it? Can we look at our own
experiences with benevolent curiosity? Can we bring that
spirit even to bad or difficult experiences, and accept that
everything changes? In a spirit of play, perhaps we can begin
to see that our own inner map and our desires exist within a
larger context, and that in fact that context sometimes
changes what happens for us internally. Sometimes, when
we place our map with another's, surprising areas open up
for exploration if we are willing to see them. What is our
intention, and can we move in that direction whole-
heartedly with no attachment to outcome? What do we
actually have control over? Can we learn to enjoy the things
we can't control while being responsible for our own desire?

Do we have an understanding of what we can and cannot control?

And finally, is there something beyond the edge of the map, the known territory? Where is that elusive bliss that we supposedly already have? We have to learn how to make do without our perfectly idealized happily-ever-after world and find a way to be satisfied with limits and imperfection.

Body

In the beginning was the word. But in our beginning we go back before the word to the thought behind it, then to the breath propelling it out into space. Even before the breath in our story is the body breathing the breath that puts the word to the thought. So we start here.

Once upon a time there was a body belonging to a young girl. What does that mean? Am I talking about her, or is she lugging around an extra body? We talk about and think about the body in different ways, but it is where we start, a bloody mess suddenly pushed out of safety with room to move and no idea what to do with it. Then the shock of taking that first breath ... But now we've gone too far. That's not where we start. We begin with the body, the physical form. In talking about bodies we think of safety, a sense of ownership, knowing this physical being as ours, feeling comfortable and secure in it. It provides a safe haven for us, and we also take the responsibility to keep it safe and healthy. We tap into the body's own intelligence, learn to hear its preferences and cope with its changes.

* * *

I sit cross-legged at the start of class. Taking my seat and letting myself settle into it, feeling all of the pieces of my day settle as well, little flecks in a snow globe gently finding their way down to rest. My muscles soften and I feel gravity take me deeper; when I feel it, I reach away from it, lengthening out of its grasp, using my own weight to help me gather

37

myself and grow taller. I am rooting down, reaching out and up, held by the earth but expanding in and out as I draw air in and release it back out. I am earth, I am air, I am water.

I love bodies, how they move, their limitations, their perfection. I particularly enjoy watching bodies move with intelligence. What I mean by that is not always that they move with grace or that they are height-weight proportional or that they are doing anything particularly impressive, although those are all fine things as well. What I mean is that you can see a body that is aware of itself and working in conjunction with all of the other parts of itself. It is beautiful to see.

Learning to Listen

One day a student told me she had finally figured out how to use her core muscles during her workouts, after hearing me talk about them class after class. She felt as if suddenly her ability to exercise productively was progressing by leaps and bounds. I told her that was always an issue for an instructor: figuring out how to say something to a student so that they can hear you and make use of the information. If you've never been in shape you don't know how to be in shape. More importantly, there is a disconnect in communication between you and your body. You don't know how to engage the muscles and pay attention to what your body is saying. Once you learn to be in shape, you can get in shape faster and keep it longer and more easily, because you know how to be in shape. If you've spent your life overriding your body's natural desires and tendencies, when you try to listen to your body, you are really only hearing all of those layers of stuff you've put around yourself. You believe your body is telling you to do all of these other unhealthy things. The truth is that your body is speaking truth—it only knows how to speak truth—but you can't hear it any more. Sex is the same way. If you've spent your whole life being told to want only certain things in certain ways, and you believe that everyone else only wants those certain things in certain ways because that's all they've ever admitted to wanting, and moreover, you believe that some higher power has written somewhere that these are the only things you can want, then that may be all you can hear when you listen to your body. Maybe those really are the things your body is saying! What defines healthy sex, like healthy exercise, varies from person to person. Or maybe you struggle because you don't really want those things, but you try really hard to want them because you don't see a picture of any other way. You may not even realize that Doors Number 2, 3, and 4 exist. Or maybe you think you want only the things you've been told to want because you've never tried to listen for anything else. In either of these situations, with physical fitness or with sexuality, if you've lost (or maybe never had) the ability to hear your body's needs and desire, you have to teach yourself how to listen and teach your body to be smart and focused on its own behalf.

Learning to listen to the body can be like facilitating a committee meeting. I think of this particularly when I'm ill with some sort of digestive upset. Oh, let's not be delicate— I'm talking about diarrhea. I know exactly what I need to do to begin treating my body, but there is a part of me that kicks and flails and shakes her fists at the sky because the treatment is not what I want. Generally what I want boils down to something simple and silly. Because I can't have it, I obsess over it.

I rarely have any sort of stomach or bowel problems, and when I do, they are usually minor and easily resolved. The resolution involves fasting, going without food or drink for 12-24 hours, depending on the severity and what I believe the cause may have been, and then drinking lots of water or herbal tea and eating bland food such as plain rice, applesauce and bananas for a day or two. My usual drink of

choice when I'm healthy is black tea, and I usually have
several cups a day. Oh, I love my tea! I feel like my day
doesn't really start until I have it. When I'm having digestive
troubles, I know it is a bad choice, so I don't have it. But, oh,
how I want it! I actually feel a sense of loss when I get up in
the morning and realize I can't have my cup of tea. It is as
though that particular cup of tea is the only one that has ever
existed for me or will ever exist for me, and I mourn it. Also,
I am resentful. Why shouldn't I have my tea? The discipline
is self-imposed; no one is making me do without tea, but I
struggle against myself as if I were my own parent or
guardian. It's not fair! Everyone else gets to have tea, how
come I don't? It really doesn't matter that I know that it is a
temporary state of affairs and that it is in my best interests
not to have tea. There is a part of me that just doesn't care
about all that. I want what I want and I want it now!

In this case listening to my body means tuning out one
part of it to listen to something deeper, literally deeper in
this case—my bowels! They know what they need and they
are talking to me. Their needs at the moment outweigh any
other votes. My point is that there are still competing voices
within me, and that it is not easy, even with compelling
reasons, to do the right thing.

How much more is that the case in a more complicated
situation? I once read a very grumpy complaint online in a
conversation about yoga teachers in general. A student wrote
in to say how much she hated hearing her teacher say,
"Listen to your body!" She went on to say, "I've had an
eating disorder all of my life. If I listen to my body, it tells
me to do all the wrong things. Instead, I have to learn to
override it." That may feel true to her, but I'm not sure it *is*
true. Frequently, listening to my body feels very much like
learning to listen to one of my pets, or to an infant. The
communication is not clear and it is not verbal; there's no
burning bush that appears and speaks to me as a facilitator
between two beings. It is much more intuitive. How do you

know when something is wrong with your dog? Maybe his breathing seems a little labored, or he's drinking more than usual, or he is less interested in his favorite toy. The longer you've had your dog and the more time you've spent with him, the easier it is to understand the signals.

When you think about it, it makes sense that listening to the body would be sort of like listening to an animal. We are animals, and our body is the most animal part of us. To learn the body's language we need to care for it so that it trusts us. We need to spend time with it so that we know its habits, its likes and dislikes. We need to pay attention to it so that when something feels off or changes we know it. We need to educate ourselves about what will keep it healthy and happy because sometimes it doesn't know any better and wants what is not good for it. By taking the time to know it, we train both our thinking minds and our bodies; we look out for cues, and when the body responds, we acknowledge it. In that way, the body is reinforced in giving particular signals and behavior and the mind is reinforced in noticing.

Thinking about the body as an animal can be helpful in another way. One trait our bodies share with animals is a certain craftiness that lends itself to survival. The ability to store fat, the ability to find more energy-efficient ways of doing things so as conserve calories, the ability to recruit other muscles or certain properties of physics like momentum to perform tasks more easily—these are all wonderful survival strategies. As a fitness instructor, I watch students struggle to learn how to override what is built into their systems. Unfortunately, these body strategies often fill us with frustration and self-hatred—anger at the body for not being the way we want it to be. My preference is to recognize these strategies for what they are and admire them for their cleverness. The body will cheat any time it gets a chance; there's no point in being angry about it. You simply have to outsmart it.

Just as with a beloved pet, we accept those aspects that aren't our preferences or the traits that annoy us because we love unconditionally. The cat throws up on your keyboard, the dog digs holes under the fence, your cockatiel hates men, your baby keeps you up all night, night after night. Or maybe our concerns are aesthetic rather than behavioral: the dog has one ear up and one ear cocked, or the cat has a snaggletooth that makes it look demented. If we value our pet (or child!), we certainly work to change behavioral issues just as we do with ourselves. But there is a certain amount out of our control that we have to work around. We eventually accept those traits as wrapped up in the wholeness of the animal. Because at the end of the day, we have a loyal and loving companion who seems to know us better than anyone else and who isn't bothered at all by our annoying little traits.

Our physical bodies can be just that sort of trusted loving companion. When we feel frustrated by something happening to us physically, or by some aspect we don't like or would rather change, we can imagine that there may be times when the body wishes our silly thoughts would just get out of the way and make space for it to do what it needs to do.

I am talking now about bodies as though they were separate from us somehow, like pets or companions, which can be helpful but is not the whole truth. We don't actually live outside our bodies, although it may feel that way when we are particularly disconnected from them or even angry at them. We live *in* our bodies.

So now it's time for a second analogy. For me, yoga is mostly about being at home in my body. We have all heard the old "my body is a temple" concept, which is beautiful but a little hard for me to relate to. I don't really want to live in a temple. It doesn't strike me as a very comfortable place to put my feet up, have a cup of tea and read a book. I'm not sure that temples are all that well insulated; don't they all

42

have drafts? Anyway, I wouldn't feel comfortable making noise there or spilling tea or picking my nose.

On the other hand, when I look around the house I actually live in, I can see some correlations with my body. For one thing, it's not perfect. There's duct tape around the kitchen faucet waiting for us to get around to switching out the back splash. We primed our spice cupboard but never painted it, so it looks a little ratty. When we couldn't figure out why it took so long to get hot water in the bathroom, we traced the plumbing on a wild and random journey all over the basement from the water heater to the sink. I opened up a switch plate once to install a timer and quickly gave up and closed it off again, trying not to think about the old wiring jerry-rigged behind it. That's just how houses are—never quite perfect. And neither are our bodies.

But our house is warm and comfortable. The eggplant exterior glows in the autumn dusk. We re-did the floors ourselves and the wood shines. I painted a tree on our bedroom wall that comforts me every night as we go to sleep. I am grateful to have a place to call our own ... as I am to have this body to live in. If I want my body to work for me, I need to accept it as is, with all its strengths and beauty and flaws. Just like my home, I can't destroy it and start over. This is where I live.

Take a Ride

Living in the body can be uncomfortable sometimes for all kinds of reasons. I come and go with my meditation practice. One day after a lull I began it again with great reluctance. I really don't like meditating, but I know it's good for me. I go through a rhythm of a regular practice for a while and then give it up when I feel even and satisfied again. But this particular time, my mind had been a stormy place and I had been getting thrown around a lot. So back I went ...

Frequently, when I have sex these days, it is in the format of a "scene." A scene is negotiated and covers a lot more ground than we often think of when we think of sex. Part of the point of having sex in a scene is to establish some ground rules and to allow the activity to proceed past the point of pain or fear or discomfort or embarrassment where our conscious, rational mind would usually end things. So we negotiate a safeword instead of using the word "no" or "stop." Our desire is to go past where we usually say no. If we cannot talk during a scene for some reason, we set up a signal and usually refer to that as "tapping out." The safeword, or tapping out, comes up when we get to a point where we feel like we just can't continue.

So this particular day, here I am doing that boring struggle you do when you meditate. Seriously, in all of these generations, could we not come up with a more creative struggle to have in meditation? I'm sitting, and I'm breathing, and I'm stuck in my thoughts. I let them go, and my back hurts, and I keep sitting, and I'm breathing in, and I'm breathing out, and my thoughts are all over the place, and I'm sitting. And then all of a sudden I come swimming up out of it with a gasp like I can't get my breath and I think, "I just can't be here anymore." My feet are getting numb and my back is hurting and I'm completely panicked. I tap out, or safeword, out of my own meditation.

Now, isn't *that* interesting? Now I'm curious. Where exactly is it that I think I can't be any more? There's nowhere else to go. So I go back to meditating.

I could say that I couldn't cope with being in my thoughts anymore, that I needed an escape from them. I think that is true. But I also wanted an escape from my body. Frequently this is how we live, in separation from the body. The body is not me; it is mine, my object, outside myself. When forced to sit in the confines of my body and come to terms with all of the physical sensations that remind me of my earthliness, I experience that feeling of fragility I'd rather ignore. Suddenly I have to think about the fact of my mortality. The fact of being physical is, I think, just a little frightening. It's like getting on a ride at an amusement park and having to ride it through to the end. It is fun, but it's also scary, and in the case of this particular ride, we don't get to talk to anyone who has already seen it through and gotten off the other end. And there are times when being on this particular ride feels overwhelming. I just want to stop it for a minute. It reminds me of how I have felt riding roller coasters, which I loathe. The few times I have been coaxed onto one out of a desire to be with my friends, I always have the sense, as the cars climb that first endless hill, that I cannot possibly stay on this ride an instant longer. I must have them stop the ride RIGHT NOW! I've seen those service ladders attached to every ride; they can stop the ride and I can climb down the ladder. I don't care how long it takes. But the ride never does stop and I do go up and over that hill and I do scream my head off and I do live through it.

And even more—I think about the feeling of almost suffocation that sent me swimming for the surface, breaking through to take a breath. It was almost a feeling of something large and spacious enclosed in too small a space, like my body was a little closet jammed full of a larger being. Whatever sort of spiritual belief anyone may have—what is true for certain is that we are made up of energy pressed into packets of matter, and to some degree our lives are constrained by the packet we find ourselves in. We're stuck here, in other words.

* * *

So here we are on this ride. We could even call it "The Material Plane" to give it a catchy title. Getting off the ride before the end is tricky. And while we can pretend it's not happening at all, like becoming absorbed in a magazine during a tricky take-off on a plane to distract ourselves, the truth of it is still present. And the thing is, the ride is fun a lot of times! Being embodied gives us so many possibilities for pleasure! It is also scary. We get hurt, we become weak. At first the pain, the injury and the weakness are all temporary. We recover and are healthy again. At some point, we encounter something—an illness, an injury—that stays with us and becomes a piece of our physical reality. Perhaps a pet dies or an older relative. We make the connection and suddenly realize we are not immortal and that pain is always with us. Getting older and dying becomes a physical reality, rather than just an abstract idea. How do we ride it out and take in all the parts of this life?

Let's look back at what happened in my meditation, because it will be useful for the rest of this book to pull some pieces out of it. First, I am sitting quietly in my own experience. That is what meditation is, but it is a skill we can choose to develop and carry with us into any activity. In yoga, we work to develop that particular skill; we present the body with an activity, or pose, and then we observe it as it reacts to the pose. In my own practice when something difficult happens in response to a pose, I watch even more carefully. As I am reacting (in the example of the amusement park ride, with panic), I observe myself with curiosity and interest. The reaction is in process but in some very important way it is not taking me along with it. I observe and I notice what's happening. My curiosity leads me to ask questions of myself: Why am I panicking? What exactly is happening? The questions are asked without judgment. It's okay with me that I am reacting so strongly. There is nothing I need to change about my reaction; I am just curious. As I ask questions, I come up with possible answers, and I run them by myself to see what resonates. As I do this I recognize several truths: there is a part of me, separate from my experience, that is capable of observing. If I can stay aware and connected to that part, I can allow my thoughts and feelings to continue as they are, neither fighting them nor getting on the train of thought for that particular ride. My awareness begins to change my experience. I'm not actively trying to derail that train, but faced with my interest, it derails itself. It gives me another choice, and at the same time it shows me how much more there is of me than just my body, my thoughts, my feelings. This is yoga in a nutshell. Remember that box I keep going on about? This is one way to look around and see something other than the box. What we practice gets stronger. If we practice seeing, paying attention to our surroundings, we can see farther.

Sex Ed

I'm about six years old, and my friend from down the street is eight. We are under my bed playing doctor. (Is this universal among children, making up these odd doctors who do such strange things as part of the exam? How do we come up with this idea over and over again in homes across the country, when it is so unlikely that most of us have experienced these things with our actual doctors?) We take our clothes off and poke at one another's nipples and vaginas. It's cold and uncomfortable and mostly just tickles. I hate being tickled. I know there is supposed to be something erotic and interesting about this activity, but it doesn't actually feel very good. We know it's naughty, and that, for me, is the most interesting part. So despite the fact that it doesn't feel good physically, each time my turn is over I can't wait to be on the receiving end again. Every time I'm on the receiving end I want it to be done with. We know we mustn't get caught, but then we *do* get caught, and there is shame and embarrassment and my adrenaline spikes.

I am at the beauty salon with my mother while she gets

her hair done, and I am bored. In the waiting room there's a ledge with magazines stacked on it that runs the length of the wall behind the chairs. I pick one up, and suddenly realize there's a picture of a naked woman in the magazine. My heart stops, or that can't really be true, because I can feel my pulse jammed into my throat beating hard. I am afraid I'll get caught, but I flip through briefly and find more naked women. That's all I have time to see. I am awake to a new possibility, that such things are available to see. I want ... something, but I'm not sure what it is yet.

I am twelve years old and at camp. I've been rooming with another twelve-year-old who seems so much older than I am. We are all able to pass for older than we are. We've already learned to dress the part and wear makeup. But this girl has a knowing air and very large breasts. She jokes with the boys and the male counselors and carries herself differently from the rest of us. At the end of the camp, the counselors have put together a slide show with photos. One is of her in profile, emphasizing her breasts. I've forgotten now, but it seems there was either a caption or a comment, something about her "outstanding features." We all laugh, but there's an ugly undercurrent. Is this something that is supposed to be seen and commented on? Later, three of us run through the halls trying to find trouble, without much success. She twines a streamer through the inner workings of an elevator door and asks us if she can tell us a secret. She's had an abortion, she says. I have been jealous of her during camp, but now I just feel sad and relieved that I am not she.

Twelve was an interesting year. Suddenly I was taller than all the other girls and gawky with glasses and red fuzzy hair. My period started, and it was nothing like those stupid sex-ed movies described. I didn't feel more womanly; I felt dirty, in pain and betrayed. But I was in my very first musical as a dancer. I felt so grown up, going to late-night rehearsals and falling behind in my homework, going over the moves with my one friend who had made it in with me.

One night during rehearsal, the dancers weren't needed but we were called, so we had to be there anyway. All of the boys who were dancing in the show were seventeen and eighteen years old, while all of the girls were from twelve to sixteen. All of us were tucked into a side room (as a side note I find myself wondering now—where exactly were these rehearsals? I seem to have a memory of a complicated combination of rooms leading into rooms into rooms.) to watch a movie. I had already missed most of it; the girls must have been off doing something else for a while. We came into darkness, and on the TV there was Patton posed against the American Flag. We all made our way in and tried to find places to sit. I ended up right in front of one of the boys who let me lean back against him. Then he began stroking my arms, finding his way down to my breasts, brushing over the nipples through my leotard. My nipples sprang erect at his stroking. He pulled me back and put his mouth over mine, sticking his tongue in and swishing it around while he fumbled at my breasts. It was hideous! It was exciting! I wanted more. I wanted him to go away. The movie was over and we all got up and left. Afterwards, I wouldn't speak to him ever again at rehearsals, although he tried to get my attention.

What did you learn about sex when you were growing up? What did you learn about your body? What are you learning now? When I think about what I learned from sex-ed, what I remember are things like anatomy: being hugely confused by the details of the menstrual cycle, trying to figure out how a penis was ever going to get inside me when I couldn't even find the hole for it, being told that sex belonged in marriage between a man and a woman and only happened when they loved one another very much. It doesn't have much to do with the reality of the sex that I have had since then. When I look at the way we (I include myself) talk about sex, it frequently has more to do with fantasy than reality. Either we act on our beliefs of how things ought to be in an ideal world—in which case we pass on to our children what we believe the best actions and responses would be in this mythical place—, or on how we fear it might be—in which case we are full of warnings and cautionary tales—or on how we believe we look to others—in which case we massage the data to make us look a little better.

In some ways this is the framework or context we create around sex for ourselves. We are born as sexual beings. I know that we often don't want to think about that or admit to it, particularly since we are—as we should be!—deeply invested in protecting children from being sexually used or damaged. Not having kids myself, I didn't realize this truth either until my friends began having them. I thought I was unique as a child, but my friends told me stories of their children exploring all their parts right from the very beginning and clearly taking pleasure from it. As far back as I can remember, I was touching myself, learning the shape of my body and trying to figure out what it all was for. Part of learning who we are and creating a sense of self is exploring the physical boundaries of ourselves.

* * *

If we are born into ourselves, why is it that we have to find our way into feeling safe in our own bodies? I get this sense that we have to somehow climb into ourselves and learn to inhabit our own bodies. How do we begin to learn that? For me, one of my strongest examples of how I find my way in comes from yoga class. I had a defining moment during my yoga teacher training. Well, I had a few. But one stands out because it was a moment that began at the beginning of my training and extended out to the end of the month.

I went to our very first early morning yoga class at the very start of training. We swept through a multitude of poses in a very vigorous vinyasa, or flow, sequence over the course of two hours. At one point we landed in Pigeon pose. Pigeon pose is a deep, hip-opening pose, done on the floor with one leg extended back and the other crooked in front.

I had done Pigeon before, but only when forced to in class. I never practiced it at home. Why? I absolutely despised the pose. And now here I am, the first day of my new life as a yoga teacher, and we're doing Pigeon. Hate it, hate it, hate it. I'm on my mat. I'm really hot and sweaty. I have no props. And I'm doing Pigeon. Only that's really overstating the matter because what's actually happening is that my body is clenching up, quivering and shaking and sweating, hovering OUT of Pigeon pose, because I have very tight, inflexible hips and I can't actually DO Pigeon pose.

That day I began what I came to call my hate mantra. It went something like this, "I hate this pose. I hate this pose. I hate this class. I hate this teacher. I hate everyone here. I hate this pose. I especially hate YOU, girly in the cute little top who drops right into Pigeon. I hate this pose." And so on. Whew! It was always such a relief to get out of it and move on to balance poses, which I CAN do.

The whole first week we did Pigeon in class and every day I did my hate mantra. I shook and sweated and cursed and hovered OUT of the pose. My hate mantra became more complex as the training continued. We were taught to allow our inner witness to watch our practice, with curiosity and benevolence and no judgment. So I added a few lines to my mantra. Now it sounded like this, "I hate this pose. I hate this pose. Isn't that interesting how much I hate this pose? I hate this pose. Why do I hate this pose? Because I can't do this pose, because my hips are too tight, and I can't do this pose. Isn't that interesting that I can't do this pose? I still hate that little girly in the cute top. Isn't that interesting? I hate this pose." And on and on like that.

One day, my hate mantra took an interesting turn. "I hate this pose. I hate this pose. Isn't that interesting? I hate this pose. I'm scared of this pose." Well. Isn't THAT interesting? Now I've got fear in there with the hate. And I'm actually really curious—why am I scared of this pose? It's a pose on the floor so I'm not going to fall. There's very little risk of injury with this pose, especially when I'm holding myself up so far out of it. I'm hooked because I really want to know the answer.

The next day in class we don't do Pigeon. We are always allowed time at the end of class to do our own series of poses and I feel a little nudge. I actually want to do Pigeon. But I hold firm; I don't allow myself to do it. This is a pose I hate and can't want to do, so I don't do it. But the next day we still don't do Pigeon in class. The nudge happens again. My curiosity wins out and I do it myself at the end of class. And I continue my hate mantra, and I shake, and I sweat, and I curse. And I watch myself and listen. "I hate this pose. I can't do this pose, because my hips are tight, and that's why I don't do this pose and maybe if I did this pose, I'd be able to do this pose."

That was it, the source of the fear. I realized that I had a certain picture of myself, a belief about myself, and part of that belief was that I was not a flexible person. That, in fact, I was a person with very tight hips. I had been doing yoga and dance for many, many years and yet despite all that I was not a flexible person. And I didn't want to let go of that because it was part of my identity, part of my belief system. If I became a person able to do Pigeon, I would have to let go of that piece of my identity and be a new person. A person I didn't know.

The next day when I did Pigeon in class something changed. My mind had opened and my body could no longer hold itself out of the pose, and phffft! I collapsed into Pigeon pose. I lay on the mat in Pigeon pose and cried and cried.

Now I'm learning how to be a flexible person with wide open hips. And I've learned something new and different about my body, something I didn't know even though I've been using this body for years now. In order to learn that, I used exactly the same sequence of observation I used back in my meditation example.

I think this is a particularly interesting example because the new knowledge came from a pose I despised, something I really didn't want to do. If I had continued to avoid the pose, I might never have learned what I did. I make this point because I extend this idea out to sex and sexuality. When we think about sex, we can kind of make a checklist: I like this, I don't like that. That's fun, but that's dirty. This feels good, that feels bad. That sounds exciting, but that sounds scary. Sometimes we stop there, take the activities from the first column and leave the second column alone. But sometimes, if we're willing to go there, the second column can teach us and open us up to the difference between beliefs that lead to patterned behavior, and truth.

Yes/No/Maybe

We can continue to follow the idea of paying attention to what's happening in the body into the arena of sex. In some ways, we are giving the body something physical to do that is deeply engaging on every level: physical, energetic, emotional, and mental. Then we watch for the response. Whatever the response might be, we can decide what we want to do with it, which might be nothing at all. Maybe we just notice it and sit with it. The inner witness watches the action and reaction in the same way a mother watches her infant sleep, with infinite patience and a sense of wonder.

Our reactions to specific sexual acts can be all over the map. There are the things in sex for which we feel nothing but enthusiasm. For me, oral sex, anal or vaginal

penetration, and spanking would be on that list, among
other things. I don't have any kind of hesitation or mixed
feelings about any of those activities, and I engage in them
with no reluctance or feelings of naughtiness or dirtiness.
But maybe you do. Maybe oral sex seems scary and
intimidating—the idea of having a mouth "down there" or of
taking something into your mouth when there are various
fluids and hair and all sorts of things to contend with. Maybe
spanking seems extreme and crazy; how could something
that hurts feel good? You have memories of being spanked in
your childhood and they completely turn you off. Maybe the
idea of anal sex seems nasty, but in your most secret
thoughts you wonder what that might be like if you had the
courage to try.

To go back to yoga for a moment, as we watch the body
move through different poses, the body itself has distinct
preferences about things. We aren't used to thinking about it
this way, but if you are right- or left-handed, your body has a
pre-determined preference for which hand it wants to use to
write and which hand it wants to use to stabilize something.
When I sit and extend both legs out long in front of me, the
right leg turns out and the left leg turns in. My body holds
those preferences in every posture I do. In fact I am right-
legged in the sense that my right leg has more mobility and
agility but my left leg is a better support and has more
flexibility. This is beyond thinking and feeling; it is hard-
wired into my physicality. We can choose to learn to do
something differently (remember, what we practice gets
stronger), but the preference is there and being aware of it
helps us. For one thing, I can appreciate the things my body
does well and, by noticing its preferences, I can capitalize on
its strengths. Also, knowing about this preference at the
physical level gives me more information to work with. Now
I know that what I think and feel about specific activities is
layered on top of what already exists physically. Some things
about my body are simply built in. I say that to make the

point that we all have different responses to the same set of activities. There is no wrong response when it comes to your own preferences. And some of the responses are complicated when you begin to consider the layering within yourself of the physical preference plus the psychology of the activity plus the emotional response. That's without taking into consideration the complex layering we receive from *outside* ourselves, from our sexual partners, our parents, our friends, or our religion. It becomes not just a simple yes or no. In the kink community there is a tradition of using a simple questionnaire for determining what activities might be fun to share. The questionnaire lists activities and then you fill in yes, no or maybe. What I find for myself is that it is just not that simple.

Let's take the activities listed above as examples. I've said they are enthusiastic yeses for me, but there are exceptions: when I'm on my period I have learned by hard experience that vaginal penetration is bad for me. There are some people with whom I just don't have the correct energetic dynamic for spanking. It feels wrong. If I don't know you've had experience with anal play, I may not want you down there. So even my "yes" is qualified.

The no's are even more interesting to me. Just look up there at the various reasons people might have for saying no to some of those activities. Hesitation—maybe I've never done it and am nervous about it. Shame—it's naughty or dirty or wrong. Intimidation—what if I do it badly? Edgy— I've never heard of it or known about it and it seems wild or nasty. Bad experiences—maybe it's connected with something else in my life, something that felt bad or went wrong or had complicated emotional context. Turn-off—it seems repugnant. Fear, embarrassment, misplaced desire. Oh, that's all interesting territory. Sometimes, when we have a multi-layered response to something, we might want to play with that and develop it a little further, rather than resolving it. Like an artist using a palette, or a writer creating a complex character, we can be the artists of our own experience and use our own reactions to color our play. There are other arenas available to us, but sex is so very clearly our adult form of play where we can allow our creativity to flow and flourish freely without passing it by an inner censor.

But this is where consent gets complicated. "No" means "no," doesn't it? Sometimes pushing at a "no" is a sexy place to play. How do we do it carefully, respectfully, staying far away from that place of assault? What does "no" actually mean?

* * *

In fantasy, I can imagine wanting someone else to take control. I can want to be able to say "no" and have that person read my mind as to whether I really mean it or not. In real life, everyone involved *must* take responsibility for the communication, even when we choose to communicate unclearly at times, and even when we choose to play in these edgy areas.

What do I mean by this? I find this hard to talk about because it is an area where I would like to be 100% crystal clear. I have been a victim of sexual assault. I have worked with victims of sexual assault. "No" means "no." How long have we worked to make people understand that? When we talk about sex, we talk about risk. The risk of pregnancy, the risk of disease. There is also the human risk of being open to one another. People need the safety of "no."

There is a "no" that is heartfelt, that says from the deepest part of my being, this is not what I want and you are choosing for me and changing my life and my landscape without my permission and without my willingness. It is always okay to say "no" and it never needs a reason.

But there are other "no's" that are an invitation to explore together, to explode what we believe about ourselves and find some more complicated truth. Exploring a "no" means the risk of changing your own landscape. Learning the difference between these two varieties of "no" is vital, and the error should always be to accept the "no" without reservation as a true statement. We need our bodies to be safe havens. For the person saying "no," you need/I need/we need to be honest enough with ourselves to find a way to *express* ambivalence if it is there. Not a refusal but a cautious welcome.

However, the beginning of this discussion carries me into a different realm beyond the physical. I have spent time getting in touch with my own animal nature and sitting with what is, learning to listen deeply and pay attention. I have spent time looking at my own sexual territory. But now I'm done with just sitting and I begin to reach out. With the introduction of "yes" or "no," something else comes into the mix, and my energy rises.

Energy

We take a breath and it's a shock, something from outside ourselves entering and supporting us. How do we even define it, without words yet? Our energy rides our breath and literally provides our inspiration. Suddenly there's something driving us and connecting us with the world around us. The boundary is no longer a simple matter of where the body ends and everything else begins. Even without touch, even without words, an exchange can happen.

We are still new to one another, learning each other's bodies. We are sitting naked on her bed with black sheets that make our white bodies almost glow, and she asks me if I know about the hankie code. I know about it, but I don't actually *know* it. It's sort of thrilling to think about this secret sexual code referring to activities I have yet to consider. She pulls out a whole set of all the colors, given to her as a joke by an ex-girlfriend, and we begin to play with them. She pulls out two (pink for breast play, black for heavy SM), ties them together and instant bikini top! I tie one around each ear to make fancy earrings. She makes a bowtie. And back and forth we go, giggling, forced to higher levels of creativity with each turn. When we run out of bandannas we pull them off one another and make love on the pile.

"Write me a story." She emails me her one-line request, and I write her back a detailed smutty story about a naughty secretary and her difficult boss and the encounter they have one night at the office party. In response I receive a memo from the boss with a reminder of the day and time of the upcoming holiday party, a warning about missing office supplies, and the ramifications of being caught stealing from the company. On the night of our date, I wear my very best inappropriate-secretary attire. A friend who is in on the game introduces herself as Beth from accounting on the third floor. When my "boss" catches up with me that evening, she drags me off by the hair, accusing me of stealing office supplies. When I stutter out a denial, she pulls out a giant-sized novelty pencil and waves it in my face, "I found this in your desk!!" And I'm lost, snickering at the silliness of it all and giddy and so wet from excitement, knowing that that pencil and I are about to get intimate.

After a lovely half-snuggling/half-wrestling session with my boyfriend, I realize later at home that I have lost my lip gloss to his couch. I email to ask if he has found it, and he responds with a picture of the lip gloss standing upright on his bathroom counter being menaced by a riot baton. In the email version of letters snipped from a newspaper, he has written, "We have your lip gloss. We require sexual favors for its safe return." I blush and giggle at the screen before sending my response, and a week later I arrive at his home to barter with my body for my precious hostage.

I show up at the club in my jeans and work boots, reporting for duty as an apprentice electrician. One of my partners is in the trades, and she has a fantasy that needs fulfilling. I spend time sorting parts for her, carrying tools and pulling wire. Part of the work requires us to use a lift, and once we're up there and she has scared me a little with the controls—jerking the lift up and down—she traps me up there with no other way down. Soon I'm on my knees with my face at her crotch, sucking her cock and begging her to let me down.

I am topping my first scene, meaning that I have planned and am controlling the action with a friend of mine. The theme is forced exercise. We are revisiting middle school PE class, the scene of much humiliation and unhappiness for us both. It feels like we are rewriting history, making it turn out the way we would like it to now as adults, taking a difficult experience and turning it around. She is doing jumping jacks for me in her ridiculous gym uniform in front of an audience, the rest of her "classmates," who have come to watch me do this for the first time. I have on my jacket and whistle. At the moment I am testing her sports knowledge; every time she answers a question correctly, she gets to move on to a different exercise. "What do you call the thing you use to hit the ball in cricket?" I ask. She slants her eyes at me, "Cricket??? Um ..." She can't come up with an answer. "Come on!" I say, "it's cricket! You've played cricket before a hundred times, haven't you? Who doesn't know about cricket?" Our audience falls into laughter at this preposterous idea, and she can't help but snicker as well, even though missing the question means more jumping jacks for her.

When our energy builds, it spills up and out, overlapping into the territory of others. Sometimes it's an invasion; other times our energy flirts around the edges of each other looking for commonality and attraction. We live inside a bubble of energy, or maybe I should describe it more as an amoeba of energy, shifting and flowing and sending out tendrils to check out the scene. When we find someone interesting, we look for ways to build energy together and keep it going. We make decisions about where to allow the flow and when to channel it elsewhere. We think about claiming our own power—our power to make decisions, define our own borders and keep ourselves safe and on track—or we choose to give ourselves over for the moment or a lifetime to another authority. In the examples above, a delicate rising energy is nurtured to connect two people and create a world where we can meet and play together. In some cases, the created world is explicit—a fantasy reality where we can act out our roles. In other cases, we are simply creating an agreement together to suspend our serious adult sides and engage with one another with no judgment on either side. We haven't made a make-believe world, but we have created a little bubble to play in safely. Once in our safe little bubble of energy we can engage with one another in whatever ways we choose—exploring fantasies, diving into specific emotional states, or simply connecting deeply one on one. We allow each other to be silly. We allow each other to be overcome. It is safe here to love and laugh, and also to be scared or angry or embarrassed or awestruck or sad. One of the great gifts of having a body is that it allows us to play with our connection to deep and powerful emotions and share it with one another.

In the Body section, I talked about just sitting and observing ourselves in action. We give the body something to do and then we watch. The interesting thing about observation is that it creates energy. In yoga classes I frequently have students do either a body or breath scan. In a body scan, we sit or stand or lie quietly and take our awareness to each part of the body individually, not trying to change anything but just observing. Similarly, in a breath scan, we watch our breath and observe its flow and how it feels. Perhaps we put words to it, describing it to ourselves. We notice which parts of our body move with the breath and which ones don't. Perhaps we take our hands onto our bellies, then our chest, then the sides of the body, then the back, and feel the breath moving under our hands. In both cases—the breath scan and the body scan—what will happen frequently is that something changes when the awareness settles. We observe. Our energy moves to follow and something changes. It's powerful stuff.

Into the Unknown

I spoke at the beginning of the book about taking my vibrator with me to yoga teacher training. I knew I would be away from home for a month and I knew I had the ability to take care of my own sexual desires during that time. Someone asked me whether it might also be a good idea to take some safer sex supplies like condoms and gloves, just in case. In this particular situation I knew there was no such thing as "just in case." I had made a commitment to myself to immerse myself in this training and I needed all of my energy for that. I made the decision to close off the channel marked "Sexual Energy Exchange with Others" so that all my energy would be available for my training. Sometimes we make a perfectly good choice not to be open and available. We choose to give our energy over to something else. In some ways, this is the definition of monogamy: we choose to put all our sexual energy into long-term life plans, into the relationship created by the two people involved. We make a choice to close off certain opportunities in order to create a particular life we want. We all make these choices whether we are conscious of them or not. If we can become conscious of them, we can perhaps make clearer choices for ourselves.

Energy is a limited resource for all of us. It's not as easily quantified as other resources, and it's not static—it can grow or diminish due to other circumstances. But eventually there is a limit. I remember very clearly learning a simple lesson in my fifth grade economics unit: If you have one dollar, you can only spend one dollar. You can spend it on a dollar's worth of candy, or you can spend it on a dollar's worth of clothing, but you can't do both. Energy is similar. Energy is not as easily measured as one-dollar bills, but the idea is the same. If I had spent my energy on sexual exchange during that month of training, I would have had less energy available for my study and practice.

Just as with that one-dollar bill, the decision I have to make with my energy is, what do I really want? What am I attracted to and what are my priorities? The funny thing about energy is that it doesn't follow the same kinds of rules as the physical body. Some things feed my energy, build it up; others drain it away. So I observe, and my energy flows to follow, making subtle shifts along the way. If I then choose to watch my energy, I can get a different level of information that will inform my choices.

* * *

So, watch the energy. What do I want? How do I know what I want? This seems like a really obvious question. I think most of us had that experience growing up of hearing about something and then trying to imagine what it might feel like and developing a desire for it. For me, kissing was first. Kissing is something that we see other people doing from a very young age. It's not considered overtly sexual so it can be talked about and done in the open (as long as you're a man and a woman, but that's a different book altogether). It is understood as a precursor to sexual activity. So I remember fantasizing about kissing. There was no one in real life I wanted to kiss, so I would imagine kissing Robin, the Boy Wonder, Batman's sidekick. There was a blank in my mind beyond that. I wasn't sure what else might happen or even if I sensed there was something else. I guessed there was, because my body had a desire for touch, although I was unable to approach that blank area even if only in my mind. My lack of knowledge and my lack of readiness created a barrier.

That phenomenon has repeated itself throughout my life. As I begin to fill in the blank areas with more ideas about what I could do there and develop a curiosity about it, I am able to somehow imagine myself doing it. Off to the side somewhere is the edge of the map again, with the blank unknown, something I can't bring to mind. There is a temptation to think about sex as something that has edges where everything stops, something clearly defined. And then within that region there are the things you like and the things you don't like. I believe it is significantly more complicated than that. Back to our energy following observation: I find some tangible thing to observe—in this case the idea of kissing Robin, the Boy Wonder—but there is a blank space all around it where my knowledge does not extend. However, if I keep my attention there, my energy flows to follow, and curiosity develops. A desire to fill in the blanks.

Back to my fantasy life with Robin, the Boy Wonder: I knew I wanted to do more than just kiss this bat-friend! So I would try to think of something else. It's funny. Children know early on which body parts are taboo. I didn't imagine Robin touching my shoulders, unless as an in-between point before reaching my breasts. Even in my mind, I would shy away from the thought. I was both drawn to and frightened by it. Gradually though, I allowed Robin to touch me. Sometimes it would help to imagine myself as someone else, so I became Wonder Woman's younger sister, Drucilla— tougher, more stubborn, more *Amazonian* than my big sis, sheltered from the world at large by my life on the island of women—a hard nut to crack by this male sidekick. He would have to be very canny to get through to me, demonstrating an interesting combination of rough desire, pursuit, and soft retreat. (Already I am beginning to determine my sexual course. In order to access my own sexuality, I have created some rules and guidelines that will become not-so-conscious triggers for awakening my interest.) I haven't even made it to the part about insert tab A into slot B, but already I've set the scene for possibilities with role play and power dynamics. I am creating the line of travel for my flow of energy, digging a channel where it can run freely.

Over time I overcome my own embarrassment, admitting to myself what might feel good or what I might want to try as Robin, the Boy Wonder, and I explore further. Oh young love! Amazingly, I never had to say anything out loud to him; he always read my mind and did exactly what I wanted, even things I was afraid to confess. I was always shy and resistant, struggling against both him and my own desire, but fierce when finally awakened.

The themes for me then about what I like and what I don't like are less about specific actions and more about the approach. I am drawn to the sense of the unknown— something I can almost, but not quite, imagine. I like to play "fill in the blanks." I like the idea of having someone show me that I want something, surprise me with it, knowing that once I'm there I can be strong in my responses without fear or shame. I like the idea of taboo, of something secret and hidden, approached with a combination of eagerness and reluctance. These ideas formed for me long before I understood the possibilities of what could actually be done.

At this point I hadn't actually tried anything yet but was beginning to taste the flavor of my sexuality.

Two possibilities with energy are clear to me now. On the one hand, by choosing not to engage sexually at my teacher training, I was restraining the flow of my energy, shutting off possible leaks in the system. On the other hand, in my fantasy explorations with Robin, the Boy Wonder, I was looking for and defining my specific desires, training the flow, sending it in a particular direction.

Pushing the Boundaries

Back to my explorations: Now that my energy is moving in a particular direction, I need to engage with another person to explore further. Robin, the Boy Wonder, simply won't satisfy my desires for long. Engaging with real people is much more complicated. Each of us sends out our little tendrils of interest, finding our way through each other's boundaries, defining them more clearly as we go as well as finding those places where our interests overlap. Commonly called flirting, this activity, I believe, is more valuable than we generally think.

But I should define my terms before I go further and give anyone ideas. To me, flirting smoothes the way, making both the person flirting and the person flirted with feel good. In my mind, if it doesn't accomplish that, it's not flirting. In yoga there is a concept of dhyana, which is a state of meditative absorption during which you align yourself with the object of focus. In some ways, flirting works from that base state of aligning oneself with the person of interest. We talk in yoga about seeing and recognizing the divine spark in each person; in this case, we actively align ourselves to that spark in another and respond to it. It doesn't (necessarily) have anything at all to do with getting some action. I tend to think of it as social lubricant.

Flirting is really allowing yourself to see another person—to find something beautiful and desirable and show it to them. I know sometimes I miss good opportunities for flirting because I am so much in myself that I'm just not paying enough attention. In that circumstance, when I look at the other person, I am only seeing myself. My energy is actually contained within my own little bubble and reflecting back at myself. I think flirting is really all about attending the moment, attending the person. My energy needs to open to that of the other person. Again I am paying attention and observing, but this time I give the gift of my observation to another.

You can see where this might get tricky. Handling and reading energy well takes skill. Earlier I talked about listening to the body on an intuitive level. Listening to energy is still pre-verbal, and now I have the added complication of having to listen to my own energy as well as that of another person.

When we desire something or someone, there's a little space between the desire and the action necessary to attain the desire. If we can become more aware of that space we can make a choice. Do we pursue the desire or do we let it go? If we allow ourselves to be controlled by desire, our energy changes, becoming overwhelming to the object of our pursuit. We are so blindly attached to what we want that we lose sight of everything and everyone else.

If we make the informed choice to pursue a desire, how do we avoid attachment to the object of that desire? In both yoga and dance, we talk about making use of opposing flows of energy. In order to jump high as a dancer, I need to push down into the floor. I get a lot more lift by pushing down to lift up. If I get too attached to the idea of going high in the air and put all of my focus there, I don't get as much lift. Gravity is a force dancers must consider; if we work with it, we can accomplish more. Learning to work with it is where the discipline comes in. That concept exists in yoga as well as in both the physical practice and in the spiritual practice. In yoga, I make a strong and disciplined effort, aiming myself like an arrow at my desire and aligning myself with the flow of forces already in play. Then I simply release myself and surrender to whatever comes.

If I just fling myself, physically or energetically, the movement is unsupported and has a frantic or flailing quality. The other piece of the puzzle is holding the center, the still point. Physically, in both dance and yoga, I can accomplish more in a safer way by holding the center, not keeping it tense or rigid but holding the awareness there and moving from that place. Energetically, the same holds true. Holding my steady and comfortable seat at the center, I am at home with myself, completely full and satisfied in myself regardless of outcome. If I move from that place, I carry my safety with me as I reach out. The corollary of that is, when I reach out to others, they can sense my rootedness and feel safe and unthreatened as well.

From a purely physical standpoint, holding the center is one of the most difficult things to learn. The problem is the muscles have to open and relax to the breath, allowing expansion and contraction. Rigidity will only end badly. On the other hand, allowing the muscles to release fully is also a bad idea. In that case, there is no support for any movement and everything becomes risky. Finding the balance takes a long time to learn, particularly when you factor in movement of the limbs in all directions, sometimes simultaneously. When I begin to look at holding my center energetically, it becomes even more complex. Now I am working with an intangible, frequently in conjunction with another person. The perfect balance is always likely to be a work in progress—figuring out how much to reach out and relax, how much to hold back and contain.

Carrying that idea from yoga with us, let's get back to flirting—that energy play between two people. When there is something specific I desire from a particular person and the flirting is more directed, how do I flirt gracefully, pursuing my desire and being clear about it, but with a spaciousness that allows the other person to move freely? Flirting ought to ease the way, but attachment to outcome feels bad to both people—the pursuer because they are desperate with their desire, and the pursued because an energetic obligation has been created without consent. So, if someone approaches me and I get the sense that I'm just the third person on their list of every woman at that event—that it doesn't matter which one of us says yes as long as one of us does—I don't like it. Or alternatively, if someone seems to be going down on a sinking ship of desperation and expects me to throw a lifeline, suddenly I have an obligation. Ick. Desire itself isn't a bad thing; in fact it's rather yummy. But don't make me responsible for fulfilling it. Or just use me to fill in the blank. When I flirt I am really approaching another person's borders. I want to do so respectfully and carefully. If someone is working a room out of a genuine love of humanity, and specifically a love of the particular humanity present for the evening, including themselves—well, that's a different situation from trying to fill a desperate void. Someone with an enthusiasm born of greatness of heart and natural exuberance rather than desperation is hard to resist. And genuine interest is hard to miss.

People who are genuinely interested in me tend to spark my interest in return, whether sexually or otherwise. It doesn't necessarily mean that anything at all will happen as a result, just that my focus sharpens. I think it is frequently true that a good way to be interesting is to be interested. Being interested in someone is another way of taking your attention there. Remember, where you bring your awareness, your energy follows. Your energy attracts their attention, which draws their energy to follow. Now you have a beginning. As a side note, if you do open your awareness and your energy to focus in on the other person, and that does not in turn bring their awareness back to you, rather than viewing it as a failure—as in, oh no, I'm a loser because this person doesn't want to date me!—try to view it as a huge success. With very little investment on your part you've discovered a place where you can safely shut down the flow of your energy in order to direct it elsewhere.

Flirting ought to make both people feel good. This requires empathy, tact and some degree of intuition on the part of the flirter—again, listening to the energy of the other person and really paying attention. There is no flirting script or correct way to go about it, except for whatever the correct way is for that particular person on that particular day. I think about the energy I send out sometimes as one of those cartoon bee swarms, the ones that all move in sync and create different images depending on their intent. Imagine the difference between the swarm shaped like a big mallet coming after you to pound you down as opposed to spreading into an inviting embrace, and you might get a sense of what would result in greater success.

When I approach someone, the first thing I focus on is that the other person is a human being, and that *I* in fact am also a human being. I am just establishing interest in them, demonstrating myself to be courteous, friendly, interesting and interested. I am creating an energetic contract with each person, asking for permission to cross the border as well as creating a space for them to feel welcomed and at ease. At this level, it would be nice if we could all flirt with one another all the time. I am holding my center clearly but staying open enough to engage and pay attention. How open I keep my little bubble depends upon all sorts of things— from my purpose in approaching to how much sleep I got the night before, to how my day has been so far, to what I expect from this person.

If my desire is for more than just social lubrication, then the next step is relaying some sense of who I am and what I like, while at the same time demonstrating that I have paid enough attention to know a little bit about what they might like. I am not trying to be something I'm not in order to get attention, but out of courtesy I do tailor what I do to the specific person and situation.

Because I don't know the state of this person's little bubble of energy (How was her day? Her sleep last night? Is he in a good mood?), I want to make sure I don't require any particular kind of response on the other person's part. My little energetic amoebic tendril is simply knocking on the door. Putting someone in a position where they have to either engage with me in any way beyond what they're comfortable with or be direct to the point of rudeness and slap me down, is not nice. I think this is where a lot of people get hung up. It really takes thought and care to put yourself out there as an offer without getting in the other person's way. Back to the idea of feeling secure and comfortable in your center—the other person needs to feel that ultimately you are good company for yourself and that they are desired but not required.

In the world of polyamory, having multiple relationship partners, I have had wonderful experiences flirting with a partner's other partners, or love interests, or crushes. It aligns me with the force of my partner's desire and creates a bond. By aligning myself with my partner's flow, I create a circle around us instead of pushing someone out. I can validate my partner's good taste and connect with them in that. I have a voice in the situation, and I choose to be supportive with that voice. Generally, I am sending friendly energy outward, and I hope, am bringing friendly energy back toward me. In that same sense, flirting can be done within a monogamous relationship with the friends and family of the other person, again aligning the energy with the loved one and supporting the bond we have. In this sense, flirting is not done as a precursor to sex but simply to form an alliance.

* * *

All this talk about bonding makes me think of my high school chemistry lessons. Remember all the little drawings of ions, how they attract one another and form bonds? There were several kinds of bonds available, some stronger and some weaker, as I recall, but they all allowed these ions to come together to form something bigger and useful. What I also remember about high school chemistry was how difficult it was to conceptualize what was happening at this very tiny level of reality, despite all of the descriptions and experiments and scale models of atoms. When we talk about observing each other and ourselves at an energetic level, we have added in a layer of complication. We can't always be sure of what we see. My relationship with Robin, the Boy Wonder, in my mind is easy; relationships out in the real world with other people are complicated.

Blowing Bubbles

If we talk about energy, we also have to talk about inertia, how to get the first push and then direct our energy. I think of inertia as a sort of deflated balloon: everything necessary is there except the air. How do you let the air in? Desire isn't enough on its own, even when it comes to sex. I want to write this book, but my wanting it isn't going to write it. When I think of that first breath of air, of energy, just to begin something, usually it looks like showing up. Meditation=butt on cushion and yoga=feet on mat; well, writing looks like my butt in my chair staring at the computer screen. Even if I'm not inspired, even if I have nothing to say, even if I don't feel like it, I am far more likely to write by putting myself *here*, than by going out for coffee with a friend, or watching TV court shows, or taking a walk. If I want to have sex, I need to put myself in a room with the person desired, and the intention must be clear for both of us.

Now that I've shown up, I need to make a disciplined effort. I think at this point people get hung up on the idea of will power. I tend to think of it more as plugging leaks. Imagine water running through a hose. Now imagine what happens to the flow of water out the nozzle if the hose has lots of leaks. When I sit down at the computer to write, I immediately want to check my email. And Facebook. And my friend's blog. Oh and that gives me an idea for something to write, but it has nothing to do with my book, so maybe I need to write in my blog. Have I received any new emails yet? Maybe I need a snack. Or some tea. The sun's out; a walk would be good. I'm leaking energy all over the place! I'm sure there are some psychological or emotional reasons for my writing avoidance, but that's the next section. Right now I'm thinking about energy. So how to plug the leaks?

Back to where we began: I pay attention to my own experience. I don't fight the leaks but I don't follow them either. I don't get angry with myself (all right, maybe I do get a little frustrated); instead I'm curious and interested. Eventually, my energy settles into the channel I've dug for it by simply being in my chair with my document open on the screen and my intention clear.

People who choose chastity are familiar with this idea. You could look at chastity as denying yourself, but you could also see it as simply directing the flow into a higher priority. I can make a decision to allow myself a purity of focus, to create that bubble of energy around myself and my desire, whatever it might be at the moment. In order to do that, I need to be conscious and directive about the nature of my desire. If I am not conscious about filling the space in my bubble with my choice, the space will be filled, but by something I haven't consciously chosen. I can see a very clear picture of this by looking out at my garden. When I clear a space in the yard, I need to plant something in the space I've created. If I don't get around to planting anything, the weeds and the other plants grow to fill the space.

So now I'm at home in my body and familiar with it. My energy has risen and begun to seek out my own interests as well as other people to share them with. I've put myself in a place to move from and created a channel to flow through. I make choices based on my energy level and on my priorities, closing off the flow in some areas and sending it out more strongly in others. I practice holding my center, feeling rooted and safe in myself as I reach out. But in order to reach out further, I need words. I need to think, I need to feel, and I need to express.

Thought/Emotion

Body and breath have had time to merge with one another when thoughts and feelings begin to arise. Can we even find the line any more between before and after when our thoughts and feelings are what give us memory? Our memory only allows us to go back so far, to the place where we began to have names for things.

I move into the mind with its thoughts and emotions and immediately my words—the ones I struggled to find when talking about the body and energy—come flowing, so quickly they spill over one another faster than I can put them down. There is a joy to this cascading verbiage; even as I struggle to contain them in some sort of sense, I can't help but smile.

I think this might surprise a few people. The mind is a lot of fun. Seriously. It is. I'm not sure we're really conditioned to believe that. I think we spend a lot of time trying to overcome things. Our bodies are one clear-cut example. There are all kinds of things we are supposed to do about our bodies, and all kinds of things we are just as clearly *not* supposed to do. Our bodies are earthy and therefore somehow beneath us. We do something similar with our minds and emotions. They are scattered, they run around all over the place, they are mean-spirited or clingy or self-righteous or proud or fearful or all kinds of other things, and we need to get them in control. We think too much or we think too little. Our feelings are too strong and overwhelming, or they're not strong enough, and we are cold and unfeeling. Our opinions about our thoughts and feelings run rampant, and the funny thing is, our opinions are themselves thoughts and feelings. How did we get ourselves into this endless loop? It seems like a whole lot of heavy lifting to get all that into shape.

I never completely bought the whole shtick about bodies being bad or unworthy or some such nonsense because it was always clear to me that living in a body was a bunch of fun. Oh, I struggled with body image and right and wrong and all that stuff, but I knew my body was all right at some level. But I really bought the whole thing about the mind. Especially once I began practicing yoga, that philosophy together with my religious beliefs at the time, and my desire for discipline and order all came together to convince me that I had to somehow rise up out of the confines of my feelings and my thoughts. In fact, I tried really hard as a child to become Mr. Spock from *Star Trek* and obliterate my emotions altogether. I did not try to obliterate my thoughts; they had intrinsic value. I just wanted to order them in a logical fashion, to *control* them. (And while I was at it, I needed to stop judging people. And make my bed every morning. And set aside a half hour for practice every morning. And walk six miles every day. And ...)

Anyway, I continued my struggle with the mind and emotions, and then I went off for my month of yoga teacher training. I discussed already the idea in yoga that each of us is made up of a number of sheaths, or bodies, that layer over one another to create our reality. The first sheath is the physical body, the second is the energy body, the third is the mental/emotional body, the fourth is the inner witness and the fifth is the bliss body. We did a little exercise in class one day at my teacher training to look at how they all interact. We were split into groups of four, and within each group one person became the physical body, one became the energy body and one became the mental/emotional body. The physical body began to move, joined quickly by the energy body, and together they explored the world around them. A little later, the mental/emotional body came along and joined in and suddenly everything got a lot more complicated. And a lot more fun. Within the exercise, I was astonished by how much I enjoyed having thoughts and feelings along for the ride. It was an awakening for me. I hadn't realized how strongly I disapproved of them in the first place, and how much work it required to rein them in.

In retrospect it's a little difficult to understand why this was a new idea for me. After all, I loved reading, I loved words and the exchange of ideas, I loved expressing myself and all of my deep feelings through my body. I respected and admired people of intelligence as well as deeply passionate people. I cared deeply for my friends. There was so much of value, and yet I wanted to do away with it all. Oddly, this aspect can become one of the entertaining parts of having this particular layer of thoughts and feelings—we can hold conflicting thoughts and emotions and beliefs all at once. Our mental and emotional layer has no trouble at all with paradox, even as it drives us crazy.

Communicating Desire

Whatever relationship you have with your thoughts and feelings, they give you tools to work with your body and the energy of your desire. Again I ask the question—what do you want? This question draws out a second question—what do you NOT want? When it comes to sex, remember I'm working with that complicated map that includes my physical being, the territory of myself, all of my thoughts and feelings about my body and my sexuality, everything I learned and absorbed from my schools, my peers, the movies, commercials, my parents, my religion, my experience. Now I take my attention to all of the thoughts and feelings that arise when I make use of that quirky, not entirely accurate map of mine.

Why is it so important to think this through? I think of it sort of like grocery shopping. We all know that if you shop with a list, you are more likely to get exactly what you need and want, and less likely to come home with that bag of chips that sounds so good in the heat of the moment. And the more specific you are, the better; if you know you need a particular brand not found in store A, you'll do your shopping at store B to make sure you get what you really want. You also avoid that experience of wandering the store, wanting something, not quite able to put your finger on it, and leaving frustrated. With sex, if you've already thought through your desire, you give yourself protection from being overwhelmed by the heat of the moment, into forgetting either your own chosen boundaries or your safety. You can clearly state to yourself and others what you *do* want, and are more likely to go looking in the right places. And you're less likely to leave frustrated because you couldn't quite figure out what you wanted.

Using my map I can look for the specifics of my desire in lots of places. I could begin with fantasy and go back to revisit the Boy Wonder once more. I began already to tease apart pieces of my sexuality revealed by the fantasy; now I look at it more closely to figure out which details specifically work for me. First, I may want to look at the fantasy as a whole to see if it is something I want to create for myself in reality. In this case, that clearly won't work: a sexual relationship between me and the caped crusader's buddy is out of the realm of the possible. If I can't have the real thing, what parts of it do I want to try and recreate? Is it about Robin, specifically? In that case, can I set up a fantasy role-playing scene with someone willing to be in costume and say things like, "Holy hotdogs!" a lot? Or is it about being with a superhero in general? Is there a particular dynamic that plays well for me in fantasy? Is it something even more specific like the mask and gloves? Do I like the idea of anonymity? Am I the damsel in distress being rescued? Or taken advantage of? Am I an evil villain being punished for my wicked ways? Am I an equal participant, fighting back with an even chance of winning? Or do I already know I want to win? Or to lose? Do I want to play out a specific story line, or do I just like the feeling of the power exchange?

Even with a fantasy that can be carried out in real life, I still want to look more closely. Some fantasies work best as masturbation fodder, remaining perfect and complete in the realm of the mind. Some fantasies are more complicated, involving more people, or props, or specific locations, or activities that might be dangerous or illegal. With every fantasy I can examine it in the same way, discarding the impossible and unethical, and picking through what's left for the details that heat me up. Is it a feeling? Is it a location? Is it a prop or costume? Is it a word or phrase? Is it a sensation? Is it an emotional quality? Is it a type of person or persons?

I take my practice of paying attention and turn it on my own thoughts, watching them with curiosity. Earlier I did a body or breath scan, looking carefully at each detail and asking myself questions, noticing how each part felt; now I do the same thing with my fantasy thoughts, digging deeper and deeper to look at them more closely.

Filling in the Blanks

I already know from my fantasies about Robin, the Boy Wonder, that at least a portion of my sexuality revolves around filling in the blanks and exploring the edges. I desire a power dynamic and enjoy the idea of being compelled to deal with things that are embarrassing or difficult for me. I enjoy the idea of playing a role. The approach rather than the activity is key for me. Now maybe I can take that a little further, look at some of my real life activities and find a unifying factor, something that brings together what I enjoy

and gives me ideas for what else I might like. I have scanned
my fantasy. Now I need to scan my mental home movies and
observe them for themes and trends, something that shows
me where I am already digging a channel for my energy to
flow through. Ultimately, I am drawing new, more accurate
lines on my map, both for myself as well as to communicate
with a lover.

I begin to pick through some of my experiences, selecting
the ones that rise easily to the top of my memories and bring
the most heat. I am not allowed by agreement with my
primary partner to have anyone else's mouth on my cunt, so
having my lover nuzzle her face against my crotch through
my jeans and chew on the seams is thrilling. One of my
partners likes to have me hurt myself for him. I bring up
strong memories of using a stun gun on my own cunt for
him, struggling to hold it against myself and push the
button, knowing how much it's going to hurt and how much
he's going to like it. I think about how many times I've held
myself open for him to beat with his belt while I'm crying
hysterically. I remember the freedom of giving myself over
completely to one partner, letting myself be used by her
friends as she chooses.

From those experiences I can pick out following rules as a
theme. Being told to do something that is painful or
humiliating works for me, as does holding a difficult pose.
Being praised for it. Even better, when being told what to do
pushes me up against a physical or emotional limit of my
own. Driving myself crazy by pushing up against the
activities I'm not allowed to do by agreement with my
primary partner is fun for me. I enjoy being a good girl, a
real rule follower, and I like to have rules to follow,
especially ones that are challenging in some way. I also like
to snuggle right up against a boundary, either my own, one
in relationship, or a societal boundary, and push at it a little.

I scan through to find more: holding hands with my
female partners in public because we're women and holding

80

hands with my boyfriend in public because I've been a
lesbian for twenty years and he's a man. Dressing high
femme in lipstick and heels at a mainstream lesbian event
where jeans and Birkenstocks are the rule. Simply being in a
long-term lesbian relationship. Having a boyfriend when I
identify as a lesbian. Screaming while I come so that
everyone can hear me and know what's happening, or being
really, really quiet while I come so no one has any idea what
I'm doing. Choking on my Top's big strap-on cock. Wearing
a big strap-on cock. Having my face rubbed (literally!) in the
fact that my boyfriend actually has a big cock. Wearing my
collar in public. Being pissed on by my Top. Kissing my
boyfriend.

This new list still seems to be about rules I have in my
own mind, only now I'm breaking them. Clearly, I like to
follow rules, but it's really hot for me to feel like I've
transgressed, that I've crossed the line and am now in rebel
territory. Also, I can see some flexibility in exactly whose
rules I am breaking; because it is exciting for me, I seek out
rules I can break in my own mind, moving easily across lines
into paradoxical or contradictory values.

Is there more? I remember being surprised by an
upwelling of heat with my partner, the urgency carrying us
into the bedroom where I end up face down with her weight
on me, crying out into the mattress, pressing a dildo into my
ass while I ride a vibrator on my clit. I think of being
grabbed by one of my Tops at a party, pulled down to ride
her thigh while she pants in my ear and I come fast and
hard. I flip through page after page of memories of being
restrained by ankles and wrists by my boyfriend and being
overwhelmed and exhausted by pleasure, by pain, by fear, so
that all awareness of limitations is gone.

Now I have added urgency and the heat of being carried
away and overwhelmed by my experience, so that all choice
is taken away from me.

Much of the heat of my desire is created by the friction of rubbing up against restrictions or limitations that are either self-imposed or have been imposed upon me. A nice feature of having thoughts and feelings is that I can make them serve my needs, twisting them in a direction that works for me, creating that friction. In yoga and in meditation we often talk about having "monkey mind." The disadvantages of being at the mercy of "monkey mind" are that the thoughts and feelings twist and turn all over the place and frequently take us along for a crazy ride, or at least fill up our heads with endless chatter. But if I am aware of that particular ability and respect it, I can harness that marvelous flexibility. Just as with the body, if I am aware of the workings of the mind—love and accept it for what it is, even as I recognize the pitfalls—I am free to play with those very aspects that challenge me. Rather than trying to make my thoughts and emotions into something other than what they are, I meet them in reality and work with them there.

Now I have drawn in a few lines on my map using both my fantasies and my past experiences, when I go to negotiate future sexual activity I can provide specific examples of what gets me wet. Some areas on my map, though, are blind spots. How do I begin to examine those? Some are blind spots because I hold certain beliefs and I alter reality to fit my belief system; others are blind spots because I find those areas disturbing in some way. I edit them out more consciously. If I am going after the truth, I need to find a way to look even here.

What If You Can't See the Blanks?

I know about both of these types of blind spots because I have plenty of them myself. I am particularly skilled at creating an alternate reality in my mind and then simply rearranging the evidence to fit my belief system. I know just how easy it is to do. It's like the opposite of science, where you come up with a possibility and then test to see if it is accurate or not. In this case, I come up with a reality and then fit the facts around it, no matter how ludicrous it is.

I have talked already about lacking a sense of direction. I also can't recognize cars, including my own. One day I came out of class and walked to my car. I tried to put the key in the door but I was having trouble getting it to fit. While I stood there fiddling and struggling with it, my eyes wandered over the interior idly. It seemed different. The locks did not extend up in view of the windows as I had thought they did. Then I noticed there were four doors. I had no idea I had a four-door car! I was thrilled because for all of this time I had only been using two of the doors. Now that I had seen them, I'd be able to use all four. I still had not managed to fit the key in the door, and it finally (finally!) dawned on me that it was not my car.

Another day I went grocery shopping. I finished teaching my yoga class and headed off to Safeway. The plan was to get the shopping done for the holidays at two stores, one for produce and fresh stuff and one for packaged stuff. Off I went on my merry way, parked in the lot and began to shop. I kept having this eerie feeling as I went through the store; nothing was quite where I expected it to be, and some of the items I thought should be there, weren't. The whole store had been rearranged, and I kept thinking it looked different, perhaps tidier or something. This particular store had recently been remodeled so it seemed odd at best that they would have remodeled and rearranged it yet again so quickly. Then I got to the milk. My sweetie likes a very particular brand of milk with a particular carton only available at Safeway. It wasn't there. And the milk was on the wrong side of the store. When I finally located the milk, I looked and looked for my specific brand but couldn't find it. Finally, I decided I'd have to get another brand. Oh look, I thought, QFC brand is on sale! Wait a minute ... what's QFC milk doing in Safeway? I thought about this for a measurable period of time. Then I started looking at the price labels. *They all said QFC!* That's when it dawned on me—I wasn't in Safeway at all; I was in QFC!

* * *

I tell these stories not to humiliate myself, but to demonstrate how remarkably easy it is for some of us to alter reality in our minds despite all evidence to the contrary. Our minds are quite nimble that way.

Another way of mentally altering reality is to simply edit pieces out. When the sister of a friend had her first baby, a boy, she sent photos to the rest of the family because they lived so far away. My friend brought one photo in to show a group of us. Her sister had done something odd. She had cut a post-it note very, very small and stuck it on the photo right over the baby's penis.

Many years later, when I began to date a man for the first time in twenty years, I was very nervous about the fact that he was a man. In my mind, I simply edited out his penis any time we got together, my own version of a post-it note over his anatomy.

I bring all this up because this is where the concept of "I like this," but "I don't like that" can get complicated. I began looking at it earlier with the list of activities for which I am unreservedly enthusiastic. Except when it's the wrong time of the month. Except when the energy is off. Except when I am with someone who doesn't enjoy that activity. Suddenly, my list of things I like to do begins to look like that spelling rule—remember the one? It goes, "i before e, except after c, except when the sound is long a, except ..." Then there's a whole bunch more exceptions. What kind of a rule is that, anyway?

Well, it's the kind of rule that actually fits pretty well with how things work. What does editing reality have to do with

84

defining desire? Sometimes something creates a physical response of arousal, but the picture we have of our reality won't allow that. Maybe we believe the activity is wrong, or that our partner won't want to do it. Maybe the fantasy involves someone other than our partner and we can't believe we might want that. In order to allow the desire, we would need to alter the picture we have of ourselves. In the case of consciously editing out pieces of our desire, maybe we think it's physically impossible or just too complicated. Or maybe we're too embarrassed to admit to wanting whatever it is, even in the privacy of our own minds. On some level we have the desire; on another level we have erased it. It becomes the elephant in the living room. We don't admit to its presence but we arrange the furniture around it.

Even with the activities for which I have unbridled enthusiasm, I still have times or situations where they don't work for me, and all of those complicated exceptions. Then I have my blind spots. I can't see them well, if at all, but I arrange the furniture of my desire around them. When I engage around my blind spots, my activities and arousal have a different feel to them. Those activities create all sorts of responses for me, everything from mild embarrassment or shame to heart-pounding fear to actual dislike. My responses have become significantly more complicated than just "I like this" and "I don't like that." Do I desire those activities? Absolutely, but the emotions around them are difficult. Again, my desire is multi-leveled and more complex than just saying that these are activities I enjoy. I may not be able to approach them directly, despite the fact that I want to do them.

And we've circled around again back to desire, trying to define what we actually want. I find myself circling this question for myself. The more I know how to define it more clearly, the more it escapes my vision. Especially since consent is such a specific part of desire. Desire can be a hunger, a driving need or vision. But for me it can often take the shape of something that looks more like enthusiastic reluctance. For others it might look like refusal forced into submission. Desire can be an open door, passive but willing, or pursuit and capture. How do we fit our ideas of consent into such a shifting framework? It really ought to be simple enough: when we desire something, we want it very much, and when we want something very much, we not only consent to it, we pursue it. When we want someone else's participation, we need that person's agreement, and with that we go forward.

Ought to be, perhaps, but isn't. We are rarely that direct in how we desire or in what we desire. In fact, we often approach desire indirectly. One method of approaching desire indirectly we learn by absorption from our peer culture. Usually it is unhealthy and unproductive. Remember all of those self-help books that tell us, "When a man says this or does that, it actually translates to some other thing"? We learn to read between the lines with one another, reading more into things than is sometimes there. And, as with communicating with the body or with our own energy, this method of communication requires a large dose of intuition. When we are misread, we respond with resentment: "Why didn't she understand what I meant?" Learning to read social nuances and to be empathic in our dealings with others is a valuable skill worth honing; using it to negotiate our sexual desires with one another, however, is tricky. It is better if we can learn to use all of those lovely words at our disposal. Approach by indirection can be very sexy, but we need to be conscious and intentional in our method.

Unlearning those unhealthy methods and learning to approach desire more honestly can take time. Remember those blind spots? If I am completely unaware that they exist at all, I find that they shape my approach to desire without my knowing it, skewing reality. Like a black hole out in space that warps everything around it but is impossible to see. As with shopping in my mistaken grocery store, I may feel uneasy or uncertain without knowing exactly why. I might need some other tools to find the blind spots and work with them clearly.

Hot Context

I am sitting in the green VW beetle belonging to the woman I am quickly coming to love. Right now love is not on my mind. What *is* on my mind is kissing her. We have been touching one another over time, flirting with the space between us. Tonight we've been sitting in the car for a long time, talking, and I keep moving closer. I have my blue shirt carefully unbuttoned to give a hint of what's underneath and I lean toward her as though fascinated by our conversation. We are right out here in public on the street in front of my apartment, and she is a woman, and oh so sexy with soft lips that move as she speaks. Finally, she leans over and touches them to mine and I dissolve in the feeling.

I am naked at a play party, waiting for my Tops to be ready for me. In the meantime, I am told to stand in front of a full-length mirror and look at myself. I am surprised at how difficult it is to do this, just stand and look at my naked body in front of other people. I am turned on but also embarrassed. One of my Tops comes over. "What do you think of how you look?" It is impossible for me to answer her, and I struggle to come up with words.

Someone grabs me right before I have to work a shift at a party, helping to monitor the space. He throws me on a futon and punches me between the legs, making me come over and over again until I am spraying come through my jeans, drenching myself. He lets me go in time to work my shift, stuck in my soaked pants that are now getting cold and sticking to my body, and now, every time I move, I am reminded and I think of him.

I have my legs tied open and he is beating me on my cunt with his belt. I can't keep myself from struggling and fighting to get away, which is why I am tied down. I can't possibly tolerate another second of this, I believe, and yet I don't use my safeword. There is a part of me recording the whole scene, knowing that later on I will enjoy it as much as he is enjoying it right now.

At a different party, my lover is gently fucking my ass with her fingers after she has massaged me into a contented puddle. As I begin to ride upward toward my orgasm I am aware of the conversations on either side of us. Both conversations are amazingly mundane and part of my pleasure is built from this odd juxtaposition.

Sometimes I can easily step outside and begin to really look at the way I've constructed my experience of reality. If I don't fit the mold right from the beginning, I immediately notice something is not right. I am able to question everything else, because if one thing is not right, how can I know that everything else is?

But even if the status quo suits me pretty well and I go along with everything because it fits me fine, sometimes I want to take a closer look anyway. Why? Because sex ultimately is an expression, not just of love or connection, but also of creativity and my ability to think a little bigger. Outside the box, you might say. Finding inspiration, seeing myself more clearly, feeding my creative juices, is valuable, and in turn it helps me find a greater range of connection with other human beings. I don't have to have sex with hundreds of people, or swing from chandeliers and read the Kama Sutra every night. I just need to use the tools available to me, to find my own range that belongs to me and my sexuality and my creativity. Sex is play, and the spirit of play needs an open mind and a following of that creative spark.

Ideally, it is a place where I can be thoroughly myself, met and matched by another or others. An exploration of just who this self might be to fully inhabit it is in order. And not just in order, but fun to explore!

Remember the fun part? I can learn how to know myself better, describe myself better, and directly speak my desire to the other person. Or, because it is sometimes less interesting and exciting to take a direct approach, I can learn more healthy ways of approaching by indirection, making use of all those funny little quirks in the map. Use the senses of the other person to help me see my own blind spots and play with them, notice those areas where paradox exists—desire mixed with fear or ambiguity or embarrassment—and use them.

That takes me back to defining those areas again. Clearly there are many factors obscuring my vision. How do I get a good enough look at them to make use of them? I've looked at my fantasies and experiences, scanned them closely and observed my own responses. But those methods might not get me close enough to the areas that are really difficult to see. I need someone else's help to take a less direct approach, sneak up on them. Another person can be another pair of eyes for me, to help me observe the external context of my experience and shift things, and to help me see myself and my desire more clearly. He or she can actually help me create context and define my own little piece of the playground more specifically. My blind spots become visible to someone else, and he or she can help me push into them and explore them.

In real estate the joke is that the three most important factors in buying a house are location, location, and location. In sex and in communicating about sex, I believe the three most important factors are context, context, and context. So much goes into determining context: the location, the mood, the timing, the atmosphere, the other person or persons, the physical state, the language, the sounds. I have mentioned

89

that I often have sex or sexual activity in the context of a scene. Just as with a scene in a play, a play scene involving sex is orchestrated to some degree. We negotiate and plan, we have a beginning and a main part of the scene, we come down from it and separate. I don't plan to talk about scene creation in detail because I know most people don't have sex in that context, and the people who do have sex that way already have many resources available to them to learn how to do it better. What I do think is relevant in this context, though, is that a part of the scene for me is to observe myself throughout and report back on what I've seen afterwards. On a practical level, this is helpful to me and my partners for pursuing better experiences. But I have also found it useful in learning new things about what I like and the complexity involved in personal preference and contextual changes. I am right back to the beginning: learning to pay attention to my own experience. Now I just have an extra set of eyes, the plan to refer back to, and an analysis after the fact.

* * *

I do things sexually that I don't enjoy at the time. They hurt or are uncomfortable or scary and I very clearly don't like it. However, after the fact, I find myself dwelling on those very activities, watching my own little internal mental movies of the action, and getting turned on. After a while I find myself asking to do the very activity I disliked again. Like my struggle with Pigeon pose, my internal struggle with whatever this specific activity is brings me up against something interesting in myself, something that rewards me in some way.

Abrasion play is a good example of that for me. The first time I tried it I was willing to do it only because I had good chemistry and a wonderful history with the person I was playing with. He cuffed my wrists and locked them to a fixed point and scrubbed me down with a stiff bristle brush all over my body, including all of the sensitive parts, while I screamed and fought and tried to get away. Afterwards, I was very clear—I enjoyed the scene itself, because it was very physical and because I enjoy this person but I did NOT like the feeling of the abrasion. Over the course of time, I found myself remembering the scene and shuddering to think of the sensation of the stiff bristles rubbing over my labia and clitoris, or stroking my asshole. I was disturbed by the memory. And turned on by it. Finally, about six months later, after a long internal struggle, I came back and asked if we could do it again. Now it is a regular, though infrequent, part of my play, something I always dislike in the moment, but the fear and the dislike of it combine to create heat. It gets me wet and ultimately that is a big factor in determining what I will and won't do. Like and dislike, desire and repulsion are less important than that simple concept. What gets me wet is what makes the cut. Abrasion is something I would never have connected with sex or with desire, so it was a blind spot for me, and the feeling of it falls into the "don't like" category. However, with the proper context, it becomes desirable.

You might notice that, in this case, I needed the help of a partner to introduce me to the idea and push me gently. I should be clear about this: I'm not talking about a lack of consent, being pushed "for my own good" into something I'm not interested in or ready for. And I'm also not necessarily talking about edgy sex; everyone has their own edges, their own places where they're scared. They vary a great deal from person to person. I certainly have areas where I feel curious but am afraid to explore. Or areas I feel doubtful about but am willing to try because of the person asking. It may be surprising to some to think about getting pleasure from doing things we either don't like or have ambiguous feelings about, but we do this in real life all the time. Most people who ride amusement park rides, or who enjoy risky outdoor sports, or who get stage fright but act in plays, or who get nervous about having too much responsibility and making mistakes but keep climbing the corporate ladder anyway, can understand the cognitive dissonance of desiring something but fearing it at the same time, or disliking what it takes to get where they want to go but doing it anyway for the reward. Pushing at boundaries as a joint effort is built in to our sex lives to a certain degree—at the beginning, anyway. Maybe as adults we forget what it feels like the first time to risk being naked with another human being, pushing past fear and pain to allow that person's body to actually penetrate into our own, or on the other hand, being the one to plunge in. Pushing together past discomfort is something we have all done at some point just in order to begin having sex at all.

This type of cooperative pushing is a lovely way to continue to explore new territory. You can see it as *almost* a part of my fantasy life with Robin, the Boy Wonder. I say almost because there was an important piece missing. In my fantasies, I wanted *him* to do all the pushing. All I wanted to do was the cooperative part, going along for the ride. It doesn't work very well that way in real life. In life we have that funny matter of consent to work around. While the fantasy of being forced into something can be very exciting and can even be brought to fruition by careful planning, when it happens randomly with no lead-in, no preparation, and no communication, we usually call it sexual assault.

In reality there needs to be some curiosity, on either side or both. Sometimes the curiosity stems from sexual desire, sometimes it's a curiosity about sensation (what does that feel like?). Sometimes it comes from fear or even repulsion. Anything that generates a heated "I would never ever do that!" has strength and heat behind it. Sometimes it comes from envy, a desire to experience something that someone else has experienced just to know what it's like. Sometimes one person is curious and the other is willing. Whatever generates it, the push has to come from both people, and it usually takes time. When I think about trying to get into a difficult pose in yoga, I don't simply throw myself into it—I work into it gradually to allow my body time to get used to the idea. Because this is an area where I may not be absolutely clear about my motivation or responses, I want to find my way carefully. It's like the difference between walking through a brightly lit room with an easy passage and a completely dark room crowded with furniture; I'm not exactly sure what I'm going to run into.

The energy to generate a push may appear or evolve, sometimes as a large wave, other times as a tiny waft of desire. I can allow it to dissipate into the air or I can begin to develop thoughts (I wonder what that's like?) or emotions (fear) about it. It may have an effect on my body (a tightness of breath, a flush of color in the face), which can be nurtured and guided or repressed and ignored. The person being pushed toward something needs to be romanced, because there is always some hesitation. I'm not talking candy and flowers, I'm talking heat. So maybe describing how hot it would be to do this or bringing attention to the physical reactions the pushed person is having. Sometimes the push is actually a pull, generating curiosity and then withdrawing, leaving the person being propelled to drive themselves forward. Because this is mutual, the person being pushed romances themselves as well. The people involved make a tacit agreement that they are in fact working their way in a particular direction. Coercion doesn't work. Sulking or threatening isn't usually sexy.

Breath play is another example for me of a blind spot area that required this particular kind of cooperation. I never fantasized about having my breathing restricted or cut off during sex, or about having my blood flow cut down. It never occurred to me to tie anything around my neck during masturbation. It simply never entered my realm of thought. When I began playing with BDSM and became aware that breath play was a popular area, I immediately established it as a hard limit, something I refused to do. I had no curiosity about it so there was no need to try it out. The idea of someone cutting off my breath frightened me, and not in a sexy way. It was much too risky to play with, I believed. A few years later I began to play with someone who enjoyed breath play. He accepted it as a hard limit for me and never suggested trying it together. We found plenty of other areas of interest and overlap. There were things we enjoyed, though, that I had never put in the category of breath play: his telling me how he wanted me to breathe, controlling my breath verbally. Hugging me so tightly it was hard to draw in a full breath. Holding my face against his shoulder so I could only breathe shallowly. Stroking my throat or wrapping his arm around my throat so my vulnerability was clear. When he stroked my throat I responded strongly and positively, and he mentioned that he particularly noticed that response. We both could have happily continued to play there, but my curiosity had grown.

I want to emphasize that last point: we had no need to explore any further in order to enjoy one another. Everyone has his or her own comfort level, and none is better than any other. I do not have to do more, bigger, faster, stronger *something* in order to accomplish what I think is the real goal of sex—connection and sharing and fun and creative freedom with one or more human beings. But for me specifically, part of my sexual interest has developed around pushing the edge, so when my curiosity was piqued, I wanted to explore it. The fact that he never pushed only made me want it more, knowing he did this with other people and enjoyed it. I wondered what it was like, what it would be like specifically with him.

Cooperative pushing can be used for anything, edgy or not, and my example illustrates the progression of events. There is the "it never crossed my mind" stage where it exists as a blind spot, the "hearing about it/seeing it/reading about it" stage that brings it to attention. At that point, whether it is dismissed completely as a possibility or embraced as an erotic desire, it remains something that takes up space and awareness within our own mental map. It may be off in an obscure corner, never to be revisited again. Or it may be front and center, large and obvious. Either way it needs a catalyst to be brought out, whether the catalyst is our own impulse, a decision to seek it out, a meeting or involvement with someone who trips or stumbles over it, or perhaps its random emergence over and over again until we can no longer define its driving force as coincidence.

Breath play and abrasion are only my examples. You can see through my examples where I am defining *my* territory of interest and desire, which will be a different territory from others. I frequently play with BDSM in a public space. I had lunch one day with a friend who said to me, "I like to watch you play because you play over here," as he pointed to the edge of the table. I liked the idea of using a tabletop to define the possible area for everyone to play in. If you imagine a tabletop as having space for everyone and for every type of activity, you can't look at it and have any sense of one location being in some way better than another. It's all a part of the same thing. Maybe you have a foot fetish, and that's all that really works for you sexually. So you play in one very tiny location on that table, never straying very far but knowing that one place very, very well. Or maybe you like a lot of different activities that fall under the umbrella of sex, but they are not edgy. There's no risk of falling off anywhere, and you have lots of fun romping right in the middle. Or maybe you're like me and you really like the feeling of fear and the unknown, so you play out where you're really not sure of your footing or of what's going to happen. Sometimes just the act of defining a larger area of interest—rather than making a list of specific activities—can open up the field of vision or create a safe place for creative experimentation. You have still defined boundaries, but everything within that space is fair game.

Here There Be Dragons

And what about taboo, playing with our beliefs about ourselves or with what is off limits? Here are the blind spots where we edit around our own discomfort or beliefs. For me there's not much that's naughtier and more taboo than peeing. Ooh, did I just say that? When I was a little girl, I was so embarrassed by this particular function, I could barely bring myself to even use the word "restroom," as in "I have to use the restroom." Any other word—toilet, bathroom, pee, piss, urinate—was completely off limits. Due to that shyness, I had many accidents, all the way up until I was in fifth grade, mostly because I could not bring myself to ask to go, you know, to the *restroom*. Even writing the words now I want to—I don't know—make the print smaller so no one can read them. The idea is still highly charged for me. I had bladder infections, one right after another, partly because it was just so hard for me to admit to having this need to pee. So it surprised me later that I began having these fantasies about one of my partners pissing on me. When I say fantasies, I don't mean the kind that happen front and center in our consciousness. No, *these* fantasies I was only barely aware of, maybe just as a quick flash of an idea off to the side before I would quickly erase them out of my consciousness.

Both my childhood experiences and the fact that this partner was male fed my fantasies. I was fascinated with his penis from the beginning. Remember the example of editing his penis out of the picture with a post-it note? In this case I had two taboos to overcome, beginning with the fact that he was male. I remember when we realized we had chemistry together. It came as a complete surprise because I had been a lesbian for so many years with no sexual interest in men. At a party we were interacting as part of a group, with our attention focused elsewhere than on each other. But we were standing close, and he began to stroke me then slid his hand up around the nape of my neck, grasping my hair by the roots and pulling me up on my toes. Our eyes met in speculation about this odd new connection. We talked about doing something more substantial about it but didn't get around to it for several years. We continued to have these little moments when we would run into each other. The first time I encountered his cock he was wearing leather shorts. He pushed me down to my knees and jammed my face into his crotch. I rubbed all around in it and when I felt him get hard, I began to lick and suck at his cock through the shorts. When we finally began to play together, I would feel its presence when he pressed up against me but never saw it or interacted with it. For me, the mere fact of his penis made playing with him edgy. Being with a man was taboo for my particular culture of lesbian America and it violated the picture I had of myself. It was a good place to push together.

We gradually worked our way toward a more direct involvement with his penis, both of us enjoying my internal struggle between my desire and my sense of self and community. Finally, he told me that in our next scene he was going to have an orgasm and I was going to help. That night we played hard with electricity, with him hurting my asshole and cunt in a variety of ways until I was played out and exhausted. We were in a little alcove making use of a spanking bench and a bed. When he was finished with me, he took off his clothes, lay down on the bed, and began to stroke his cock. He had me kneel over him so my breasts hung down over his penis, and he began to jerk off against them. After a little while he said, "I want you to hold your weight on your right arm on my chest so that your left hand is free to fondle my balls." I was excited and terrified, wanting to finally touch him but still in denial about the fact that he was, in fact, very much male. When I worked up the nerve to touch his balls, he groaned slightly and began jerking off faster. With his other hand he reached around and stroked my cunt, finding me dripping wet. Embarrassed, I looked up to meet his gaze. He was looking down at me in surprise. Until that moment I don't think he really knew whether this little experiment was going to work with me or not. Would I be so bothered by his maleness as to turn cold? The tricky part of working with taboo is that it can easily trigger a negative response. In this particular case, my desire for him as a man, not just a Top, was now evident to us both. All of this went through my mind and I felt the communication between us as we looked in each other's eyes. And then he slid a finger into my ass, and I was back in the moment again. Time was moving as I rocked to an orgasm, breasts beaten by his hand and his cock, stroking his velvety balls.

With this first taboo we worked together to explore an area that was both frightening and fascinating to me. Sometimes it can be part of the fun to gather the courage to ask for something taboo, especially when it is difficult to talk about at all. Remember how I had trouble even using words about the act of urination? In order for me to fulfill my fantasy I needed to pull myself together and ask for what I wanted. I was hideously embarrassed to confess to it, but that became part of the excitement—letting him see my embarrassment, being exposed. When we agree to partner with someone in an intimate way—however we define that and whatever it means to us—part of what we provide each other is a safe space. We may play with concepts that feel emotionally explosive but we always do it in a way that allows the truth of the other and welcomes them in. In this particular case, my request was met with a gleeful and grateful response. The next time we got together we played hard and long, and frequently through the scene he would drink a big swig of water and make a show of checking to see if his bladder was full. Finally, at the end of our play, he suggested it was time for a shower. I realized he did plan to piss on me and my reluctance to do something so new and scary and shameful came out again. I don't know that I said anything in particular, but he could feel my hesitation. He said, "It will be all right. It's no big deal." That calmed me enough to follow him into the shower. He had me take my clothes off and sit on the floor with my legs spread, looking up at him and finger-fucking myself. I looked up into his face and then down at his cock, aimed at my stomach. It was a frozen moment, long enough for second thoughts but not long enough to do anything about them, and then I could see the stream of piss flowing and feel the heat. I looked back up at him, surprised and turned on. It was really happening. He told me to fuck myself and I could feel his urine pooling up in my hand and then being pushed into my cunt. It was erotic and intimate and beautiful.

In these examples we gave each other a context of safety within which to explore taboo, allowing our responses to be what they were, rather than predetermining them by our beliefs or our fears. Because we shared the experience, we become witnesses for each other as well, adding a new perspective.

Reflex

Another realm where we can find information about ourselves is in our patterned and conditioned responses to some stimulus, whether it is an idea or something seen or felt. We all have kneejerk responses that are fertile territory for exploration. However, highly patterned and conditioned responses are often almost invisible to us because they are like reflexes—they bypass the thinking brain and simply react. Yet another blind spot. Our best opportunity to catch a glimpse of them is often after the fact. Once more, we simply watch with benevolent curiosity—Wow, this happened and then I reacted in that way. Isn't that interesting? The social aspect of contemplation can come into play by enlisting another person to watch with us and draw our attention to what they see. Often another pair of eyes can see what we miss. Maybe there is a visual cue, like erect nipples seen through clothing or the moment of anal penetration, that triggers a rush of blood to the genitals. Maybe in conversation something comes up, like having sex in public or pissing on someone, and we blurt out, "I would never do that!" Once we see it and take our attention there, the energy follows, and we can make a determination of what we actually think about it, given the consideration of our thinking brain. If we have enlisted another person in this pursuit, they become part of our context.

While I think of context as the room in which the action is taking place, it also refers to a depth of knowledge and mutual understanding between the players. I recently joined Facebook in order to connect with family and old friends. I told my current local friends that they were not my first priority for this particular social networking form. However, what I have found is that Facebook almost requires high context. In other words, anything I might share with people who no longer know me is either inconsequential or requires a lot of explanation that is too lengthy for the format. Regardless of my intentions, the form simply works better to keep me connected with my current friends who know me better, and so know my context more thoroughly. I have friends who joke about doing "no-context theater"—in the sense of making statements that can only be understood with the background information—but they are really referring to extremely high-context theater.

When we begin a sexual relationship of any sort with someone we begin to share context with them, even if it's only along the lines of "I really like what you're doing right now." As a relationship continues we begin both to share our stories with each other and to create a story of our own. However, there are places where we assume shared context without confirming it. Being in relationship with another human being is an opportunity again to explore those parts of our map that we've never questioned. Our eyes slide over that particular piece of landscape: it is how it is and it will always be that way for everyone. It's a reflex. When we feel that way about something, again it has the effect of vanishing into the background. It seems so clear and so obvious that it needs no discussion. Until we bring another pair of eyes and another brain attached to another body into our realm and they take a look around. Having that other person can help us observe more closely and bring more attention and awareness to our blind spots. In my house at the moment, I have any number of things that I simply don't see anymore because they have faded into the background. When I have visitors, suddenly all of those things pop back into view. We can give one another that gift of vision for our own interiors as well.

* * *

My partner grew up an athlete, loving sports and working to excel and compete in them. I grew up a non-athlete, loving books and my own company. Somehow we both came to a place of body intelligence; we just got there in different ways. As she and I have talked about our unique experiences, trying to find some common ground, I have realized that the sentence I wrote above—"I grew up a non-athlete, loving books and my own company"—is not the complete truth. Now that I have her eyes on my story it simply doesn't hold up.

And this is the thing—we tell our stories the way we've seen them in the past, and the way they've been told to us by everyone around us. This was my story: I was a non-athlete. I hated sports, loathed and suffered through PE and had to be forced into going outside to play. But here's the rest of the truth: I began dancing at age five, loved it and wanted badly to excel. I danced around my bedroom, creating lengthy choreographies to Barry Manilow albums. I played Chinese jump rope with my friends until it was too dark at night to see the rope. I'd lazily ride my bike or skate around the neighborhood. It was a joy to walk in the spring and enjoy the trees. I began observing my family early on, watching how they handled their health, and I began to make my own choices about how I wanted to live in my body. When I started practicing yoga at twelve, I fell in love with the deepening relationship with my own physical self. Now, as an adult, I spend most of my working time in a gym teaching physical fitness and loving it. It is not so much that my first story was wrong or that it wasn't true; it simply, once again, wasn't the whole truth. And I was not able to see the part that was missing without another person listening to the story with me. What a gift we give one another, not just the opportunity to witness another person's truth but to be granted deeper access to our own truth through their vision. None of my own sexual discovery would have been possible without a partner to explore with me.

What is Sex Anyway?

So I have a partner and we're exploring together, and I'm kind of curious: just what is sex anyway? Some of the examples I've given above probably don't sound much like sex to a lot of people. In many ways it is more about something happening in my head than a physical activity performed with a partner. We all come up with strange definitions along the way, and some stick with us, whether we are conscious of them or not.

On my third date with my first real boyfriend, I found myself naked in his bed. I use the passive voice for a reason; I did not think and decide along the way to end up there. I simply followed suggestion and there I was. Isn't this how it often happens for many of us? We don't remember ever choosing something; instead, we simply end up somewhere. We are shopping without a list. We can choose to learn how to create a space between impulse and action so that our actions are more carefully chosen. But nonetheless, I was seventeen years old, and there I was, naked in bed with a boy who was also naked.

I was very glad to be there, don't get me wrong. When he touched me in all of those places I had longed to be touched, and then I realized that I could also touch *him* in all of those places that were so very different from mine ... Well, it was thrilling. I was so shy, so scared to let him see me, and also so curious, sneaking a peek when he got up to change the music to watch his butt as he walked across the floor. This was the beginning of a grand adventure. From there, we tried everything we could think of (which in retrospect wasn't a lot because we were young), but it was a good beginning. But we never had sex until many months later.

If we never had sex, then what were we doing? We would kiss and fondle each other, he would stroke me to an orgasm, or I would do the same for him. He is the boyfriend in the story whose father walked in on us during our first blowjob together. It was a little longer before he ever put his mouth on my sex. I couldn't bring myself to suggest it so I had to wait for him to come up with the idea. But no sex! Not yet.

Later on in life when I worked in the sexual assault field, I realized that this is a very typical teenage definition of sex. Sex is only sex if an actual penis goes into an actual vagina. Otherwise, it's something else that is not-sex. As adults it is a little easier to realize that this is a limited definition of sex. Most parents would have the view that everything we were doing in that bed was sex and probably would have had a lot to say about it if we had been their kids. Luckily our parents were unaware.

This is an example of an obviously limited and limiting definition of sex. And perhaps even a little dangerous because if anyone had ever asked us, in the interests of safety concerns, if we were having sex, we would have, in all honesty said "no," without really understanding the question. What is sometimes harder to see is that we continue to limit our definition of sex as we get older. We expand it (maybe) to include oral sex and anal sex, but we still think primarily of a limited list of activities involving the genitals. Usually it requires two people, so we don't think about having sex with ourselves, or with more than two. And we still think in terms of insert tab A into slot B, rather than paying attention to what is happening internally.

One yoga workshop I took specifically focused on poses to help support the female body during menstruation. First we talked about things to do to support the body before it begins to bleed, and then we spent a lot of time doing restorative poses addressing the discomfort or pain of cramping and body aches that often attend bleeding. It was two hours of attention on supporting the reproductive system and everything that comes from that. Most of the class was spent lying down in these very restful poses. And yet by the time the class ended I thought I was going to die if I didn't have an orgasm. In fact the first thing I did when it was over was to go into the bathroom and masturbate. So I don't know—was that sex? It felt a lot like it to me. Along those same lines I have come out of dance or yoga classes feeling so full of physical vigor and emotional good will that I felt I could make love to anything in my path, whether animate or inanimate. When I was in Costa Rica doing my yoga teacher training, I often felt like I was making love to the ocean when I went out to swim. I have had conversations in person, on the phone or over email that caused my blood to rise and my pulse to pound.

Is sex an activity that only includes very specific things from a checklist involving body parts we cover up with swimwear in some way? Or is it something we feel? Or is it a continuum of feelings and behavior and activity?

From the example above it's clear that many teenagers arrive at a definition of sex that is severely limited. They don't create that definition out of thin air. What are we actually explicitly taught about sex? I imagine we all took away very different pieces of information depending on how old we are now, what region we grew up in and what was covered in sex ed at the time, what our parents chose to share with us and how they did it, and what we found out through our own explorations, snooping around.

As part of our sexual discovery, defining ourselves and our boundaries along the way, we create blind spots. When we define something, anything not in that definition will be excluded. If we can forget about defining the activity of sex so specifically, then we can use our skills of self observation to notice when something makes us feel sexy or aroused, expanding the definition of sex and opening up to more possibilities. Then we don't have to feel bad or wrong or guilty if we don't enjoy those more mainstream sexual activities that we are supposed to want. We also gain more possible avenues for arousal and sexual connection. When some possibilities are closed to us, we have somewhere else to go.

* * *

I talked earlier about doing a body or breath scan, really moving through each part of either the body or the breath and paying attention. Then I scanned through fantasy and experience. At this point, we are almost doing what could be called a sheath, or layer, scan. In every physical activity, as we become more proficient, we get better at mentally running up and down the body. Are my feet solid and hip's width? Is my tailbone lengthened? Is my belly hugged in and lifted? Are my shoulders relaxed down the back? At the beginning, the list of things we have to keep track of is overwhelming. Who could possibly pay attention to

everything at once? As we become more skilled, we realize
we *don't* pay attention to everything at once. We just
incorporate the questions and we constantly quiz the
different parts of ourselves. It becomes second nature. Now
we can become more skilled at scanning through all of our
layers as we examine our sexuality, venture out and
experience more and more. When I do this activity, what
happens to my thoughts? How do I feel? Am I embarrassed?
Do I feel differently afterwards? How does my body feel? Is
it tense and yet swollen and hungry? Is my energy spiking
high, or drained? The Inner Witness is awakening.

I am paying attention to myself, becoming an explorer of
my own landscape, both inner and outer, and I've invited
someone else along to enjoy the ride and keep me company.
We show ourselves to one another. We aren't just navel-
gazing together, though. There is a larger world out there of
which we are a part, and a larger framework containing us.

Witness

Look. Touch. Feel. Imagine. Breathe. React react react. Finally, quiet, and a separation. I amuse myself, I entertain myself, I annoy myself. I watch myself and I am moved. I feel tender toward this odd little person. But who is this "I" anyway, watching me?

If we were all left in innocence to explore ourselves and one another in a perfect world, I have no idea what sex would look like. I probably wouldn't need to write this book. It's easy to sit here and wish I could live in that magical place, but the truth is, it is so far outside my frame of reference I don't know if I would rather be there than here, or not. It's like trying to imagine that I grew up differently from how I did. Maybe it would have been better, but I also would have been a different person. That different person might have looked back with the very same "what ifs" I have now. And I like who I am, which leaves me to make peace with my own frame of reference.

I also recognize that my ideal world will be different from someone else's ideal world; the values and beliefs that make me shudder in disbelief may be the very ones you believe the world needs more of. From the moment we are born, our framework is being built by where we are born (both time and place), the social norms of that space, and our parents' intentions toward us—sometimes wanting the best for us and already making plans for how to create our future, protect us, and teach us what they have learned, or at other times, damaged themselves, our parents damage us in turn, warping our growth. We grow up and learn, have experiences, talk with our friends, and watch TV—either accepting or rejecting each piece of data about sex and our bodies and ourselves without recognizing that, whether we accept or reject an idea, by reacting or responding to it at all, we have already allowed it into our landscape, and the territory is shaped around it. If we ever saw it at all, we stop seeing it as it becomes normal. It becomes one of our blind spots.

It's difficult to put a value judgment on this shaping. Maybe we grow up feeling that some activity is particularly shameful. That feeling could destroy a relationship, or it could make the sex really hot, extra sexy because of the taboo. We may not be able to reshape our sexual territory, but we can look closely at what made it how it is, really look at the landmarks and draw ourselves a better, clearer map. Then decide how we want to use it. Do we want to avoid certain places because they seem too dangerous? Or do we want the adrenaline rush of extreme sex? Do we want to explore some areas by talking with friends or our lovers or a therapist? Or do we want to create a fetish of desire around it? Everyone will have a different take on it. Each landscape is unique and what you choose to do with your map will be as well. Your choices in the past may have been blindly guided by others in your world, but now that you have a map, you can choose your own direction for your very own reasons. Your choices may not be my choices but that doesn't matter. They belong to you, as mine belong to me.

I keep coming back to this idea of forming a safe place to play together. I believe that when we come together in love and intimacy, we are practicing our yoga together. Yoga in the sense of what the word itself actually means, yoking together, becoming something larger and whole. In order to do that, we need an agreement. We agree to be present and witness one another. In other words, we leave our beliefs behind and we simply watch what actually happens, the reality of it—physically, energetically, emotionally. We agree to leave the inner censor behind. Play requires freedom of creativity and a sense of permission. Even more, then, it is important not to allow any other form of censorship within our safe space. All of the societal attitudes we've absorbed need to stay behind. This is our private place together. Bullies, keep out! No judgment, just curiosity. Isn't this interesting what happens when we do this together? We agree that when things go wrong, we still hold one another in love and safety, observing and learning from even the mistakes we make together. We make a space together that is safe from the intrusions of the outside world.

Sitting in Community

I'm working a volunteer shift at the local sex-positive club, making coffee and putting out snacks to prepare for the party. One of the men who attended the orientation is following me around. We don't usually allow people to hang around between orientation and the party to give ourselves space and time to set up, but for some reason I've since forgotten we made an exception. He is eager to help me, to talk to me. He asks about what I'm into and whether I have plans for later. I can feel the waves of hunger coming off him and I struggle not to push him away.

Later at the party, as I work my shift and wander around to talk with people, help new people feel comfortable, I get several more invitations from needy men. I recognize the hunger. They are filled with a secret need, something they've kept hidden for so long and that it is hidden even from themselves. They know that they are hungry, but they have forgotten what they hunger for. They see me but they don't know me yet. They don't know themselves. They are being devoured by the hunger and are desperate to be rid of the feeling of being eaten from the inside out. The only thing they can imagine (Can they really imagine anything right now? Only the hunger is real) is that eating someone else might somehow ease the suffering, fill them up.

What interests me is that many people come to this club believing that the mere act of changing their venue will heal them. But this hunger is something no human can satisfy. Searching for something to feed that hunger is a losing proposition. In some way, though, they are right to come here, because here at least they will find people who are interested in sitting with sex, and with everything that attends it and its desire. We talk about sitting in meditation because the idea is that we literally just sit and observe ourselves. Frequently people go to places where they can meditate together in a group. I recently came across a rather novel idea for me, which was that contemplation is not necessarily a solitary pursuit, that in fact contemplation requires people working together as a social unit. Our larger social unit has created this strangely unhealthy and untruthful concept of sex and sexuality. Maybe by forming a new social unit committed to observing itself more clearly around these issues—thinking about them and sharing insight with one another—we can deconstruct our old unhealthy ideas.

So here among this community, perhaps these men can sit with their hunger long enough to allow it, understanding that, once they begin to pull out their more concrete earthly desires from the overwhelming yearning, they are among people who will be able to see them and accept them and help them achieve their desires. You know that funny little map we've drawn over ourselves and lived by? If it is too far off from the reality of the landscape of who we really are, it creates a feeling of invisibility, of being unseen and unrecognized. Even we have a hard time seeing it ourselves. It just feels wrong, and more so over time, until the hunger overtakes us. We have no box to check off and we want it, we yearn for it. I believe it's a hunger to just be who we are, a hunger no one else can feed. With a chance to just sit with it and observe it from our center, with other people holding space for us with their own heartfelt desire to be with the person we really are, we can relax into the hunger rather than having it drive us blindly.

I believe that people want to connect with one another. We want to know each other in some way. We want to create something bigger together, whether it's an intimate life-sharing relationship of some sort, or simply building bonds together as a society that help us get along, creating an easier flow of life. The easiest place for us to do that is to begin where there is shared experience. But what happens when the supposedly shared experience is exactly what defines you as different?

* * *

One day in class, I sat at the front waiting for the last few minutes to tick by before I began to teach. Sometimes during that time I stretch or center myself; sometimes I take it as an opportunity to chat with students. On this particular day about fifteen students sat on their mats, waiting for class to begin. One of my regulars sat close to me up front. She asked me if I had any children and I said no. She glanced from my face to my left hand where I wore a ring on my fourth finger and asked, "What does your husband do?"

Her intention with these questions was just to connect, to know me better and begin to create shared experience. She couldn't know that her first question set off my radar and made me cautious, while her second question brought all my walls up and put me on full alert. To her, the questions were simple. To me, the questions were a minefield. Do I answer them honestly, and, if so, to what degree? Knowing that any degree of honesty will out me in some fashion to my entire class.

As I tell this story, I can see that this is really about my desire for control. I don't want to be pushed into telling the truth, the whole truth and nothing but the truth. I want to tell the truth on *my* terms. I want to choose the time and place—the ideal moment. In response to her questions, I reinforce my boundaries against her. When I think about the energy boundary around myself, I think of it like the membrane around a cell in the body—it is semi-permeable, so it keeps some things out and lets others in. The difference is that I am in control to some degree of how permeable my membrane is, whether consciously or unconsciously. If someone hurts my feelings or I'm frightened, I may seal myself off more fully without really being aware of it. If I'm engaged and interested in someone, I will open myself up more fully.

Situations like this frustrate me intensely. I want so much just to connect and to do it honestly. When people reach out to me, I want to reach back. I think back to my energy bubble, or my amoeba, or my cell membrane again and the economics lesson of one dollar in hand meaning one dollar to spend. My energy, everyone's energy, is limited to some degree, and we make choices all the time to open up and let the energy flow or close the valves and keep it contained. Sometimes energy flowing out of me is a leak—something draining me that needs to be plugged. Sometimes I allow energy out because I know it will be fed back to me and become a feeder rather than a leak. No one else knows the status of my own personal energy system at any particular time except me. That makes me the decision-maker; I am completely responsible for my life and the priority choices I make. I cannot possibly make a rule for myself or for anyone else about what I must do in any given situation. Which means that every time it comes up, I will need to examine it, carefully examine myself, and make a decision. I dearly WANT to control the woman asking the question, I WANT to control the culture that has created the assumption of each person's reality, but the truth is, that little bubble around myself, that one-dollar bill I have, is the only thing I can control.

Practice Makes ...?

So, if this is what I have to work with, then I want to work with it as skillfully as possible. I want to know it. The more clear I can be about the truth of myself, the more easily I can move from my steady center to respond to whatever comes. I want to keep my center engaged but open in response to what comes from the world around me. When I am asked for truth, I need to give myself room to breathe, just like holding my center in yoga practice. I don't want to tense automatically in reaction, closing myself off. I also don't want to lash out off center before I have a chance to observe my own energy and desire of the moment. How do I do that? What do you think? I practice, practice, practice ... and teach myself to move skillfully.

As a yoga student, yoga instructor, and teacher of other styles of physical fitness, I've observed both in myself and others the desire to practice only what we're already good at. Sometimes I watch students who are not fit and who do not have a history of working with their bodies try to move through particular exercises. If they have a natural body sense, they do just fine. Other times I watch them come up with alternatives that simply don't work. Either they misunderstand the point of the exercise and come up with an inappropriate replacement, or they believe they can't do it so skip it. Occasionally those students will approach me with their frustration; they work out regularly, they complain, but they aren't losing weight or getting fit. Well, that's because they aren't actually working out. They show up, which is the first step, but they aren't really paying attention to what's happening, and they allow themselves to fall back into their normal patterns instead of challenging themselves with something different. If you ever studied elementary school science, you may have spent time watching tiny creatures under a microscope. Even those small beings move toward pleasant stimuli and away from unpleasant stimuli. Look how little brain it takes to move toward pleasure and away from pain! Even with a bigger brain we humans have the same tendency. Doing something we are good at feels pleasurable, and usually we are very good at doing things that are habitual. Our bodies are accustomed to certain ways of moving. When we try to move differently, our bodies are uncomfortable and try to get back into a more habitual pattern. Similarly, we are accustomed to interacting with others in a certain way. If something comes up to interrupt that pattern or challenge it, our first response is to move away or move back into a comfortable patterned response. Our patterned response complicates our search for the truth of our desire in any given moment. Ideally, we would not respond automatically at all, but instead just sit with what is happening for a moment.

What we usually do, just like those tiny creatures under the microscope, is move toward pleasure and away from pain. It makes sense to do that from a survival perspective, but not so much from a desire for skillful action. What was the last new activity you tried? Were you good at it immediately? Were there parts of it that were hard? If we can't see an immediate benefit, or if we're not extremely motivated, it's often hard to see it through. Here we are back looking at desire again, this time trying to sort out what we *think* we want from what we *really* want. Because sometimes pointing ourselves in the direction of our desire is difficult, and we need to be really clear with ourselves about it.

If I think back to the hunger of the men showing up at my club, I can recognize it because I have felt it myself. What do I mean when I say I need something I can't get from what I currently have in my life? What do I actually need that I am not getting? If it's only sex, as in a physical activity leading to orgasms, I can masturbate perfectly well by myself. So what's the problem? But that never seems to fill the need that I feel. In fact, sometimes it just makes me need more and more. If I talk about my partners filling my needs, it is almost as though, like the men in the club, I want to devour them whole and fill myself up with them. Or maybe as though I'm putting together a puzzle and trying to make the pieces fit to form a particular idealized picture I have.

But what is it specifically that needs filling? Is it only an empty space without form, voracious and grasping within me, never fully filled or satisfied? Or is it a space with a particular shape requiring a particular something or someone to fill it, if only I could define "it" well enough to find that specific thing?

Is it that I don't feel sufficient, that I need someone to either complete me or to fill me up somehow? Maybe to build me up, make me feel real? What is it that happened with the Velveteen Rabbit? He was loved into being. Is that what I need in order to be real?

Is it about the sex, or am I just afraid of disappearing? Maybe I know the map I have isn't quite right, and I don't feel completely seen, even by myself.

I have heard the idea that needing something is really a call to the divine, because neediness can never be satiated by anything else. If we can fill ourselves from that well, then we truly are loved into realness by an endless loving source that sees and pays attention to us always, allowing us to be a something all on our own.

Filled with the divine and aligned with that energy, I now have room for simple desire, something that can point me in a direction but which allows me to choose to follow.

So again, what do I really mean when I say I need something more? In my mind, that feeling is attached to a yearning of hope in the beginning of something, followed by the work and the disappointment of returning to human reality—in other words, the world of limitations, where gravity holds me to earth and I can never live forever. I yearn for the divine, the ideal, free of limits. But here on earth I learn to love despite the limits, freely.

Limits

All right, so here I am stuck on earth in this limited physical realm: what are the limits I work within? What are the pieces I can't control and how do I work around them? And how do I cope with change, both around me and within me? And again I ask: what do I want?

Being honest with ourselves about our desire can be complicated. Sometimes we feel a desire but hold a belief about that desire that is untrue. In many spiritual traditions there is a concept of sympathetic happiness, the idea being that we can learn to rejoice in someone else's pleasure, regardless of our own circumstances. It really isn't far off from feeling empathy for someone else's problems. I have noticed that I sometimes have what I call sympathetic envy. My sympathetic envy can create a false understanding of my own desire.

Back in high school when I had my first serious boyfriend, we began to share our pasts with each other. As he told me about his adventures hiking and scuba diving and sky diving, I was overwhelmed with envy. I couldn't believe he had already done all those things. I wanted to do them, too! More importantly, I wanted to have already done them. It took me a long time to recognize that I had no desire to do those specific activities; those were his dreams, not mine. What I actually envied was the sense of adventure I saw in his history that I believed was lacking in mine. I wanted the sense of adventure, but my adventure needed to be defined differently from his.

Now I lead a fairly settled, average-looking life, but I have found my own sense of adventure in two areas—my sexuality and my physicality. Sometimes we are fooled into thinking we want something when we don't. When feelings of envy arise, we have to be careful to recognize specifically what the envy attaches to. Otherwise, we may find ourselves chasing someone else's dream.

Sometimes we have conflicting desires. The students I mentioned earlier probably have a heartfelt desire to lose weight and get fit. However, I would guess that they also have a heartfelt desire not to do what is required to get there, as well as a heartfelt fear of change. Most of us feel that way about something. I may have a heartfelt desire to experience sex with a man, but if I am in a monogamous relationship with a woman, it's going to be complicated for me to get there in an ethical way. Sometimes it just looks like too much work: I really want to get from point A to point Z, but do I really have to go through the alphabet to get there? I need to decide which desire is stronger and then be willing to cope with the consequences. Either stay where I am and be content, or make the change and accept the disruption of my regular life.

In every case, I am brought back to paying attention. If I don't pay attention, I might be sent off sky diving for my desire, thinking I want to do what my boyfriend did, only to realize as I am about to jump that I don't really want to be there. Or I may be confused or depressed because I don't seem to be getting anywhere, when the truth is that my desires are pushing me around in directions completely opposed to one another.

I am back to the problem of defining things. Once I have defined something for myself, I can no longer see anything out of that box. By building the box, I have "banished" anything that exists outside it, very much in the way that I feel "banished" myself from the boxes other people have created that don't include me. I had a student in one of my

classes who talked about that idea regarding exercise. She
had not exercised for most of her life, and when she finally
began, she noticed that one difficulty for her and for others
was how to get past thinking, "I can't do that." She said the
temptation was always to walk into class, look at what was
happening and say, "I can't do that," defining the activity as
impossible and thus "banishing" the possibility of adapting
it. Then the next step was simply to walk back out and give
up. In fact, if you are flexible in your thinking, you can
always look at an activity and say, "I can't do that exactly,
but I can try this, which is similar." What you look for is the
purpose of the exercise. Once you know the purpose, you can
come up with other things that fulfill the identical purpose,
even if the exercise looks different from the original. Our
little monkey minds excel at this sort of thinking if we only
give them enough information and the room to move.

We need to find that still point at center, where we are
not fighting or following our own thoughts and feelings on
auto-pilot, as well as not fighting or following automatically
what comes in from outside ourselves. If we find that still
point and pay attention to what happens, we have a good
start. I think we also need to give ourselves room when
thinking about desire, to know that sometimes we just go off
in the wrong direction, recognize it and turn around.

Sick and Wrong

When you fantasize, who are you in the fantasy? Really
think about it: are you yourself or a fantasy figure? Or do
you surprise yourself when you really give it some thought.
Maybe you are the other person who is doing something to
you in the fantasy. Maybe you're watching it all unfold.
Maybe you are everyone present. When you read erotica or
watch porn, who are you? Do you put yourself in the picture?
If you're a woman, do you stay the woman? If you're a man,

do you stay the man? Is it hard for you to imagine yourself in it even as you are getting off on it? Are you secretly watching and the sneakiness is part of the turn on?

In sex as well as in life we make assumptions without any particular basis, and go on without examining them. So if I fantasize about myself with Robin, the Boy Wonder, I might assume that I am myself in the fantasy. It seems reasonable, but what if it turns out that I'm picturing myself as Robin, seducing this innocent young thing?

We make other kinds of assumptions as well. When I first began exploring kink, I ran into the idea of play rape as something people enjoy and practice. I have been raped myself and worked in sexual assault for years, so when I heard about play rape, I made the assumption that I would be disturbed by it, that it was a bad thing to play with in fun. What I found in reality was that my body, my mind and my emotions are all perfectly capable of distinguishing between the real thing and something close to it done for fun. It didn't bother me at all as it turned out.

We also have community assumptions that we adopt as our own. When I first came out as a lesbian, the region I lived in had a very strong lesbian presence. That particular community also had very strong opinions about what was acceptable and unacceptable sexual behavior. It was interesting to spend some time in that, because in a way, it was a microcosm of how we all live our lives. In that particular community the specific quirks were thrown into high relief by the fact that our community itself was not mainstream and had beliefs and values that went against our larger culture as a whole. Common values are easier to see and question when strongly contrasted with others that are different. An example is our culture of corporate America where we accept that men have to wear ties with their suits. No one really gives it a second thought, other than wanting the tie to be a particular length or thickness, depending on the fashion of the moment, and having the color and pattern suit the outfit. Beyond that, we don't play anthropologist and wonder about the purpose of men dressing up their necks with a strip of cloth. However, if you transplant someone from another country who has a different cultural imperative and who doesn't wear neckties, suddenly you become aware of that person's difference. Perhaps you also become ever so slightly more aware of the strangeness of neckties.

Back in that time and place as a new lesbian, the rules of my community were sometimes strikingly different from the larger context I came from. As a lesbian, I wasn't supposed to do anything "male-like," so penetration during sex was bad. Remember, as a teenager my only definition of sex was vaginal penetration by a penis. When you look at these two concepts thrown into high relief against one another, you begin to suspect that our ideas about almost everything are determined by who is around at the time. Even my fantasy life was curtailed both by the lesbian community and the feminist movement. They both dictated that if I fantasized about certain things I was supporting patriarchal, misogynistic, and sometimes racist structures.

Remember from my examination of my own experiences that I like to follow the rules and be a good girl? But which rules do I follow now? I keep running into conflicting values of right and wrong sexual behavior. My larger culture is telling me that I can only have sex with one man, and in fact that the only sex that counts is when a male penis enters my vagina. My lesbian culture is telling me I can never use vaginal penetration for sexual pleasure. I am also supposed to control my fantasies to conform to social norms. I also may make my own assumptions about the beliefs and values of the people I meet. I get nervous about how I look to them. Where do I fit when none of the rules seems to work for me? When one set of values or assumptions comes up against another, we can feel uncomfortable and judged. How often though do we actually create our own feelings of discomfort, by acting as judge and jury for ourselves? Do the rules truly originate from an external source? Or do we sometimes create them for ourselves out of our beliefs about what everyone else must be doing and then try to navigate by them? Do others really disapprove of us if we step outside the boundaries or do we create the disapproval, feeling central to our own worlds? I need to go back to my center, living thoughtfully, ethically, paying close attention to my choices, and trusting my own conscience to guide me. Instead of assuming what will work for me sexually based on something I see outside myself in the culture around me, I need to look inside and follow my own heart.

Change Never Changes

It's hard enough to follow an inner compass in areas where the path is clear. We form and follow ethics to a greater or lesser degree depending on our nature. But even in those areas where we understand that our happiness depends upon being true to our hearts, we make choices all the time to move against our deep desires. Sometimes it is fear guiding us, sometimes we allow other desires—for status or money or security—to override the voice of the heart, or sometimes we start walking one day down a particular path and forget to look up every now and then.

In sex and sexuality our guidance systems themselves lead us astray. We lose sight of what we want because we are in training from childhood to incorporate the systems around us. We try to follow the system of the rewritten fairy tale, the one with the happy ending and the clearly defined characters. It is so uncomfortable talking about sex *at all*, that talking about sex truthfully in the face of the fairy tale is close to impossible.

What happens when something in your desire shifts or changes, something that you believed defined you? What happens when you're afraid? What happens when you desire or love where you shouldn't? What happens if you don't desire where you love? Or if you don't love where you desire?

* * *

As a child I was a very picky eater. I had five vegetables that I would accept on my plate, and I ate peanut butter and jelly sandwiches for lunch every single day. My parents and teachers—and later in my teens, my friends—tried to change my habits. I fought and I struggled and I kept my eating habits. Much later, I found myself drawn to foods I had avoided as a child. Other foods began sneaking their way into my diet in very tiny quantities or in very specific places. My tastes changed in substantial ways.

I still think of myself as picky, and I think by most people's standards that would still be true. But sometimes I catch myself saying, "I don't like that," when it's not true. It was true once and it is still part of my inner landscape—such a kneejerk response that the sentence reaches my mouth before I have a chance to reconsider, even after the truth has changed and become something else.

It seems reasonable that this would be true not only with food, but also with lots of other things. Most of us have had a similar experience of changes in preferences over time. How we think and talk about ourselves lags behind our actual experience, but eventually we catch up.

Why don't we believe this might also be true of sex and sexuality? And even of gender? I wonder if the answer is partly social and political. I came out as a lesbian while in college, and for many years that truth about me defined my social structure and often my political reality. Those of us who claim an alternative sexuality have reason to be wedded to the permanence of our own definition, because we struggle to achieve our rights and recognition within the larger community. When my relationship structure expanded to include a man, not only was my own identity suddenly in question, but also that of my whole community. It makes it look as though we can pick and choose, and if that's the case, then we ought to pick and choose the correct thing, right? I imagine that even my family is invested in my lesbianism: now that they've accepted it and my relationship, how dare I go and change things? (This is not their question to me; rather, it is my question to myself in their imagined voice. I am creating my own discomfort without checking the reality of it.)

I realized the other day that I feel threatened when the people around me change. It doesn't matter how close I am to them, I just don't like it. Once I have them established in my mind as one thing or another, I don't want to have to rearrange my internal furniture. It makes me cranky.

I'm the same way with myself. If something is going to change I want to be on top of it, in charge of it. It just doesn't always work out that way. Change just *is*.

How do we separate out the different layers of changes in biology over time, in our own ideas of what feels good, or in our following along with what we are told?

* * *

I am twelve or thirteen years old. I have been using pads for my periods but they are bulky and they leak. My mother suggests tampons. She tells me how to use them and I lie on my bed and try and try and try to put one in. It hurts. It feels wrong and awkward. I can't really believe that there is any hole there large enough for what I am trying to fit. I think ahead to the possibility of sex, which I know involves putting something even larger into this (for me at this moment) non-existent hole and I am scared that I am defective somehow. I will never be able to have regular sex because I'm put together all wrong. I am a failure because I can't be a woman the way I ought to be, can't even use a stupid tampon.

I am seventeen years old and I am in love with my boyfriend and we have a wonderful heat between us. We have been trying to get his penis into my vagina and so far it hasn't worked. It hurts too much. I'm too tense. I still have never put even so much as a finger inside myself. I am still not entirely sure that I have anything down there that will hold a penis. He and I have a lot of fun anyway doing everything else we can think of and we keep trying. And finally one day, he is on top of me, pushing, and I am under him, pushing back, and I can feel him begin to pull back, not wanting to hurt me more, and I gather my courage and determination and push my hips up hard against him and there he is inside me. I am shaking and holding him close so he can't see my face because suddenly I am shy about this feeling of exultation rolling over me. He slides in and out of me slowly and cautiously until he reaches his orgasm, fearing that I am hurting and overwhelmed, but the truth is I just feel joy, joy, joy!

The joy of vaginal intercourse for me becomes over time the feel of another body pounding into mine, both of us slick with sweat and breathing hard, more of an athletic endeavor for me, but with a teammate for whom I am rooting strongly. I want his pleasure so I can ride it. For me usually the pleasure of orgasm comes earlier doing other things. This part is my gift to another.

Until when I am nineteen or twenty my body begins to struggle with it, reject it. A penis sliding into my vagina has become agony, sandpaper rubbing my most sensitive places, waiting now for his release so that I am free to run to the bathroom for cold water to rinse myself, or even better, ice to cool the inflammation. Twenty years later, I can look back and understand that my little microclimate down below, my own little ecosystem was out of balance. Some organism or other is growing too quickly and some other too slowly. Something is out of whack, but I am still too young and too inexperienced and too shy about using the words and asking to know. To me, it is failure again. My body has something wrong with it.

So when I feel the shift of an internal dial moving from an enjoyment of both boys and girls, to a passionate focus only on my own sex, I am relieved to discover that the particular lesbian community I am to join now frowns on any sort of penetration. I can let go of this particular athletic event with no regrets, and do only the things that bring me pleasure.

And then ten years later I am revisiting my struggle with tampons! This time it is a little rubber cup I am trying to use. I lie on the floor of the bathroom, covered in my own blood, wrestling with this tiny thing that looks sort of like someone cut the handle off a plunger. While I battle with slick fingers to fold it up and insert it, I recite my mantra, "I have had sex with a man; therefore I can insert this thing!" I am truly grateful to have the experience of intercourse in my memory to hold on to. This time around I *know* I have a hole down there large enough to fit this damn thing.

Later still, fingers have begun to find their way back in again, and toys occasionally. I can't pick out the moment of stepping back over that line, but once I take the step I find something surprising. Over time, my body has changed its mind. What was once beautiful only for the connection and the gift of pleasure to someone else has become a pleasure for me. And not just pleasure—heart-stopping, throat-wrecking, pounding, spraying waves of heat. Literally spraying as I discover when being fucked for hours by five different women. Sore and exhausted near the end, I have lost count of orgasms numbering over fifty, when one of the women comes back for more. She thrusts her cock deeply into my angry cunt and then pushes me away in my leather sling, arms and legs spread wide, and I swing back through the air and am again impaled on her. As I swing back off and pound back into her hips again, I feel an ocean current moving within me. The wave overtakes me and suddenly it is real, salty, and wet, drenching her cock, her pants, spraying out over the floor. My body has learned to squirt, to ejaculate. I am screaming and crying, "What the fuck is that?!?"

After that my body wants everything it can take inside it, pounding, heaving, greedily gulping it all down. I understand finally vagina dentata, the vagina with teeth, because mine has become ravenous, devouring everything in its path. How did this develop from the shy and reclusive hole I could never find? It has given birth to itself, finally, in an ocean of sensation.

My body, my body, my body. I'm not saying me, I'm calling it mine. My belonging. My object. But it defines me. And I limit it. I still don't understand it completely after all of these years. It keeps changing or sometimes my perception of it changes around it. Sometimes I am so grateful for it. Other times I feel betrayed by it. I wonder if it sometimes feels betrayed by me, by my niggardly praise, by my reluctance at times to treat it nicely, to take care of it.

Today it's my knees. They have wrinkles, you see. The skin is beginning to sag there, just over the kneecaps, and it hangs in tiny folds. I do not care that I am fit and healthy; the skin is aging anyway in its fit and healthy way and it sags. And I just want to cry. What is happening to me? The fear and sorrow I feel are overwhelming for such a tiny thing. I am scared. I don't want to die. Oh, I know I'm not dying right now. But in a way I am dying every minute and there's the proof of it in my saggy knees. I don't want to lose what I have but I know I will. It is the biggest, hardest breakup there is: the universe is breaking up with me, just letting me go into nothingness. My body is breaking up with me, dissolving into ash.

Feeling so much difficulty with aging is, well, difficult! I ought to be better at this. I should be steady, facing the changes with open arms and a loving heart, looking to the future and satisfied with the current state of things. Instead, I just want to cry and stomp my feet. I want every surgery there is, every cream, every pill, every lotion if it will let me keep what I have and give me back what I've lost.

And there's the bitter truth of it. I am not some sort of higher being, easy at all times in all circumstances. My thoughts and feelings throw me into a fever, a tempest, following every assumption, encouraging the seeds of insecurity, pushing away what I do not want to accept in myself.

And what I do not want to accept is that I am not calm. I am not at peace. I am raging, fearful, anxious. I am tossed in a hundred different directions, and I cannot find the still point.

It is odd how even while I feel I need to recognize and acknowledge this truth, I am still also cooking lunch, thinking about the things I need to get done, checking email. I am not sure if this is healthy or not. Surely I shouldn't just wallow?

But I do think it might be good to sit and watch this for a while. Every age has its collection of traits, but they do change. We lose one, we gain another. How can we not wish to personalize our own little basket of traits, like ordering from a menu? "Yes, I'd like the feeling I have of comfort in my body now, but with the skin from my twenty-year-old self, please. With a chocolate shake." With *that* skin, over *these* muscles, I'd be just great. Or we look ahead to what we think we will become, not realizing that something will be lost along the way. We think we can keep it all as we go, just adding on to what we already have. The truth: we never really get to have it all. We are not really in control.

Creating Heat from Truth

Here's the fact of it: things change and I can't control them. Well crap. So now what? All of us run into those things in life that we can't control. Okay, we can't control most things in life. We want so badly to have control over every aspect of our lives and we struggle with it to greater or lesser degrees off and on. Sometimes we think we can control things, but we are mistaken. In yoga there is that concept again of approaching life with both effort, as a direction of will and of desire, and surrender, letting go of all attachment to outcome once we have come to terms with what we want. So we come back to those steps again: 1) Define the desire, 2) Point yourself in that direction with all of your heart, and 3) Let go. In the yoga pose called Warrior 2 we embody the archer, taking aim with all of the strength we have available and then releasing like an arrow, in a specific direction but at the mercy of the atmosphere.

In sex, we run into the same issues around control and they can create a lot of distress. Maybe we desire someone or something we can't have, or at least can't have yet, and we suffer for it. But if you can't control it, you can't control it. We create our own suffering by our responses to those things out of our control. We can choose to fight them, or just accept those things. Or we can choose to make them hot and sexy, which is a lot more fun.

* * *

But before I move on to fetishizing delay, frustration and delayed gratification, I want to make sure I've actually done all I can to point myself at what I want. I have always had a hard time admitting either to myself or to anyone else what I really, truly desire in the deepest part of my being. Why is that so difficult? I'm so scared that I might not get what I want, that I might fail to achieve or to receive, so it just seems easier not to want anything at all. In some ways, I have been encouraged in that direction by my studies of yoga and Buddhism and philosophy. For other people, perhaps their deep belief in God and an afterlife has a similar effect. I end up with the idea that I should deny my body, deny my desire, purify myself by letting go of what I want. For me there is a secret feeling of relief in that idea. It feels safer somehow to let go of desire. I know that I used those teachings to convince myself that staying safe in my little box was the best choice, the most spiritually mature choice really. If I am honest, I confess that it's terrifying sometimes to think I might get what I want. My whole life would change.

When I got together with my primary partner, I was twenty-three years old. I felt like I had a lot of sexual history and experience behind me (I know, I know, don't laugh), and it seemed reasonable to tie myself to this person exclusively for the rest of my life. And, in fact, she and I love each other deeply and live together well. We both strongly value commitment and have both a desire and a curiosity to find out what it's like to move through life with the same person. But by the time I was in my late thirties it was also apparent that there were areas that didn't work quite so well for us, and that I still had desires that spilled outside the bounds of what we had established. Our culture is very specific about what is allowed in that circumstance. We can make do with what we have, distract ourselves with other things and learn contentment with what is. We can leave the person we are with to try and find a different person who will somehow miraculously encompass all of our needs. Or we can cheat. While our culture frowns on cheating, it is nonetheless one of the allowed responses within the framework that has been established. The poorest choice certainly, but a choice. We have to think outside the framework to find other choices.

My choice, our choice, was for me to seek outside my primary relationship with the knowledge of my partner. Our first attempt was catastrophic, as we could have expected trying something new without any role models or support or history to be. When that failed, I moved on. I still remember a day sitting in a coffee shop with a friend, someone I liked very much but didn't have any particular romantic draw toward. However, she had particular skills and knowledge in BDSM that I wanted to experience, and it seemed safer to play with someone I didn't love or want so desperately. My first lesson in negotiation, in voicing my true desire. There we were, sitting out in public, having coffee, and she asked me, "So, what do you like? Spanking, flogging, caning? What sounds like fun?" My face flushed and I wanted to evaporate. I couldn't imagine having this very explicit conversation about sex and desire right out in the open. It seemed crazy. And what does that say about how I, how we, have learned to communicate about sex? That the very idea of having this conversation was out of my realm of imagining.

Learning how to do this, knowing the desire, expressing it clearly right out loud are all things we must learn. What we choose to do with these things is an entirely different matter. And how we react to what we choose is another thing again.

* * *

But let's assume that we have recognized and stated the desire. Now there's something out of our control. Maybe we have to wait to get what we want, so time is a factor. In my primary relationship, trust was an issue in going from a long-term committed monogamous relationship to one in which I was free to roam. For my partner to feel safe, my freedom needed to be restricted in some way. I felt a little like I could suddenly see a whole world outside my gate, but now I was being told I could only take five steps out of it in either direction, and call first, and only in certain clothes with certain people, and only on every other Thursday, and ... well, you get the picture. Freedom was within reach, but it was being taken away from me the minute I began to taste it in tiny little bites.

Remember being a child waiting for Christmas or summer vacation? It's almost beyond endurance, isn't it? Feeling the time pass so slowly. The adults around you seem oblivious and uncaring, you can't imagine that you will survive that long, but finally the time does come. I remember almost the exact moment that I realized this truth about time; it passes regardless of desire or dread. I lived in an apartment building with three other women during my last year of college. During our final month of senior year we all felt completely overwhelmed by stress, by everything that had to be done before the year end. At the same time, we were anxious both to be out and done with it all and to devour every second leading up to the end, because we knew this was the end of this particular experience for us. We each made a huge calendar of that final month with all of our commitments and posted them on our bedroom doors. Each day we crossed one day off the calendar. As time went by, no matter what we had done, accomplished, or left undone, the day was always crossed off at the end of the day. Exams were taken, papers were written badly or well, classes ticked off the time until the end, but every day one more day was marked off. I felt a giddy sort of freedom, knowing that I could run away, sit in a movie theater for hours on end, do anything I wanted and still that day would be marked off at the end of it. And that, while my decision to blow off my assignments would have an impact on what happened to me in my life, my life would still continue even in the face of that. That realization made it much easier to simply sit down and do the work.

I feel the same way about sex and boundaries; I am always left with the choice to do whatever I want. I am responsible for my own choices and actions. No one is making me do anything. I might feel trapped, but that is an illusion in my own head. I am completely free. For me, that makes it much easier to simply follow the rules and to make the choice to get some pleasure out of the things I can't do.

How can you possibly get pleasure out of something frustrating, something that you can't have, or at least can't have yet? When we sit in meditation, we begin by finding it almost impossible to just sit quietly with our thoughts. There are a variety of ways of helping ourselves out. One method is that when a sensation comes to our attention, maybe a lower back tweak, we pay very close attention to the feeling, as well as to our own responses to it. Maybe the feeling begins as a vague discomfort, but as we take our attention there, we feel a burning. Perhaps it begins to pulse as we get anxious and want to do something about it. We feel restless. Maybe the pain begins to spread out or center down into one tiny point. Whatever happens, the point is that it shifts and changes and we move right along with it.

We can take that a step further when feeling frustrated about having to wait for something we want very badly. We can pay close attention to exactly how much we desire this thing, and in particular to how our body physically changes when we imagine being able to have what we want. How good it will feel. The anticipation of the good feelings merges with the frustration to become pleasurable. It is no less frustrating, just as with that child waiting for summer break. But now the frustration itself is pleasurable, or at the very least interesting. Remember, we observe with curiosity and interest, so what we observe becomes curious and interesting. Still frustrating, but so inextricably linked with possibility that it now feels good in some way. The wait creates more time to build the anticipation. Even if we aren't sure whether we will get what we want or not, the desire feels good in itself. We begin to understand that time passes, that our desires change or shift, or sometimes the world shifts around us to bring us a new opportunity, and that everything will be all right. Everything *is* all right. Somehow we relax into joy right where we are, without a need for anything to be different from how it is.

Bliss

*My body is limited and vulnerable. I live in it, accepting
it as it is and wanting the very best for it. I feel my energy
pulsing, my breath moving energy in from the world
around me and expelling what I no longer need back out
into space. I can allow myself to be seen and known and
held with no requirements. I can know that I am wanted
here, that there is a desire reaching out to me, pulling me
into being. I can think and feel and still understand that
there is a quiet place of rest within me. I can play for the
pure joy of it, allowing my limitations to feed my
experience. I can make a habit of joy.*

My lover is on her belly, naked, lifting her ass to me as I
thrust a blue dildo into her vagina. Earlier she was giving me
suggestions, "Wait ... a little slower. Now just the head." Now
though she is beyond that, crying out as she comes over and
over again, and I ride along with her, thrilled by her
pleasure.

I am sitting in my partner's lap after playing, enjoying the
physical closeness. We have been playing for over a year and
have known each other even longer, but tonight I feel like I
am really seeing him for the first time. He keeps poking at
me, tickling me, and I squeal and giggle, then turn to look at
him. I can't get enough of looking at him, and in my mind I
hear over and over, "So this is you! This is you."

My partner and I are at a friend's house and I am tired
and ready to go home. The conversation shifts to hair and
how to take care of it. Before I know it, we are all three in the

friend's bathroom and she is washing my partner's hair while I sit sleepily in a corner watching my partner be cared for lovingly.

I am sucking the cock of a new play partner. He looks down at me and says, "You're a good little cocksucker, aren't you? Your boyfriend taught you well, in his kind and gentle way." I snicker around his penis, choking a little and trying to keep going, despite the ridiculous idea of my kind and gentle boyfriend. I look up at my friend and feel the connection with both him and the absent boyfriend, and I know I am loved.

Bliss is that final layer, or sheath, in yoga philosophy. We are in it already; it is part of us all the time. Don't get me wrong here; this is not about looking on the bright side, or finding the silver lining. When I get a good snit going, nothing bugs me more than some little Mary Sunshine trying to cheer me up. It's more about finding that still point again. We live in limitation, we live with time passing and bodies changing and people coming and going. Our thoughts and feelings move around constantly. That still point at center is constant, always there, always wanted and drawn into being by whatever brought us here. We don't have to look for it or pretend to be something we're not; we just have to know it's there through everything else. And how do we know? Practice, practice, practice. Practice just letting things be the way they are, even when they suck. If I want everything always—my body, my society, my energy, my culture, my partners, my friends, my thoughts, my house, my everything—to be different from what it is, and struggle to *make it that way somehow*, no wonder I'm exhausted all the time! That's a whole lot to set myself against. Instead I go inside.

In a way, we can think of our lives as improvisational works of art. If you have ever been involved with improvisation, in music or theater or dance or art, you already know that it is the limitations in part that help create the art. If someone tells you, "Make a piece of art!" you may feel stuck. What kind of art? Painting? Sculpture? Should it be big or small? When do they need it? Should it be abstract or a still life with an apple? But if someone gives you just a few constraints—a realistic oil painting—suddenly it begins to take shape in your mind. And if you're given many constraints—a realistic oil painting of an apple in fifteen minutes—you are forced into creativity, especially if you don't know how to paint. We are being forced into creativity right now. We live in limitation. We all get sick and die, our bodies have individual quirks that hold us back in some areas and pull us forward in others. We can't get into someone else's head or body, so we are forced to learn to communicate across a vast gulf. Our energy ebbs and flows. We want more than we can ever have and we feel so strongly. That shape of reality is what gives us the freedom to create our lives. All those things above that I want to change somehow—force into a particular shape—are exactly my tools to work with to create my art. We are so terribly fragile, but so strong in our ability to work with that.

Go make some art—a life, say, maybe about so long—filled with love and friendship and pleasure, and live happily ever after.

Resource Guide

As I have mentioned, one of my great passions is reading. I could not possibly list all of the books and authors here that have influenced my life, even by narrowing the field to the topics of sex and yoga. However, there are a few that I would recommend highly that have particular relevance in the context of this book.

Yoga

The Wisdom of Yoga: A Seeker's Guide to Extraordinary Living, by Stephen Cope.

Stephen Cope explains with wonderful clarity the basic tenets of yoga philosophy laid out in Patanjali's Yoga Sutra. His writing is warm and very human, full of personal stories, so this ancient spiritual tradition feels completely relevant and accessible without losing any of its complexity.

Self-Awakening Yoga: The Expansion of Consciousness through the Body's Own Wisdom, by Don Stapleton.

This is the book that led me to choosing the Nosara Yoga Institute for my yoga teacher training. Frequently people think of yoga poses as set in stone and handed down for thousands of years. Don Stapleton honors the beginnings of yoga as self-exploration, experiments done by setting tasks for the body and paying attention to what happens next.

Meditations from the Mat: Daily Reflections on the Path of Yoga, by Rolf Gates and Katrina Kenison.

Written as a year's worth of daily thoughts and meditations following the Eight Limbs of Yoga, this book is funny and inspirational and honest, and an easily digestible beginning text that gives a sense of what exactly these yogic principles are.

Wheels of Life: A User's Guide to the Chakra System, by Anodea Judith.

While I never explicitly refer to the chakra system in this book, I use the system all the time as a structure for approaching my life. In a way, the origins of my book were in a yoga workshop I taught for a while called "Sexy Yoga," which was based on using yoga poses and the chakra system to create comfort in our bodies and ease with our sexuality. This book is one of my favorite resources.

Eat, Pray, Love: One Woman's Search for Everything Across Italy, India and Indonesia, by Elizabeth Gilbert.

Hmmm, is it yoga? Well, I don't really know, but I do know that the author's very personal quest for truth in her own life resonated strongly with me. While she doesn't specifically explain any of the philosophy of yoga and meditation, she is wonderfully descriptive of her own healing experience with the tradition and practice.

Meditation/Buddhism/Other spiritual practices

Loving-Kindness: The Revolutionary Art of Happiness, by Sharon Salzberg.

And honestly, everything else she's ever written. I believe I was most influenced by this particular book by her, but I would recommend all the others as well. Her writing is clear and simple as she takes on different aspects of Buddhist philosophy and meditation practices.

Open to Desire: Embracing a Lust for Life, by Mark Epstein.

A slightly different take on desire from within a Buddhist perspective. Epstein explores the idea that while desire may be a cause of suffering, it's not necessarily bad.

The Spiral Dance: A Rebirth of the Ancient Religion of the Great Goddess, by Starhawk.

As with Sharon Salzberg, I would recommend anything Starhawk has written. While my book doesn't particularly refer to paganism or earth-based belief systems, I believe strongly in the sacredness of our bodies and our energy, as well as our connection to the earth and its natural cycles. Those beliefs inform my writing, and Starhawk is a wonderful author with whom to explore this territory.

BDSM/Polyamory/Alternative Relationships

***The Ethical Slut: A Guide to Infinite Sexual Possibilities*, by Dossie Easton and Catherine A. Liszt.**

***Opening Up: A Guide to Creating and Sustaining Open Relationships*, by Tristan Taormino.**

***SM101: A Realistic Introduction*, by Jay Wiseman.**

***Sensuous Magic: A Guide for Adventurous Lovers*, by Pat Califia.**

***Different Loving: The World of Sexual Dominance and Submission*, by Gloria G. Brame, William D. Brame, and Jon Jacobs.**

When I began to list books in this category, I ran into some trouble. The books that have had the most impact on me are specific to my life, my sexuality, and my relationship choices, and they have also changed significantly over time. As a child, I was influenced by the particular books about sex given to me by my parents, as well as by anything I found or happened across by accident. In my twenties, I read books primarily relating to lesbian sexuality, history, and relationships, as well as large amounts of feminist theory. More recently, I have read more books like the ones listed above in a category pertaining to polyamory, power exchange and kink. I have never really read books about sexual technique or about creating healthy heterosexual relationships, although I have certainly read some excellent books on creating healthy relationships, period. I know there are many wonderful books out there on all of these topics. I have chosen to list the books above because 1) they are excellent introductory texts into BDSM, polyamory and alternative relationship forms, and 2) those areas are perhaps the least familiar to readers, and these books are some of the most helpful in understanding the concepts I talk about in my book if you decide you want to explore further.

And one more resource that's not a book: The Center for Sex-Positive Culture in Seattle. This is where my own explorations into BDSM and alternative sexuality began after my first experiment in polyamory went kablooey. The people at the CSPC have remained part of my community ever since. If you don't live in Seattle, I'm very sorry. The CSPC hosts workshops, social events, support groups and play parties and is a warm and welcoming environment in which to explore your desires.